CRASHING THROUGH WALLS

A Memoir of One Family's Life After Traumatic Brain Injury

Janis Ruoff, Ph.D.

With Contributions by Jeff Bouck, TBI Survivor

www.janisruoff.com

ISBN 978-1-943650-31-6

Library of Congress Control Number 2016947579

Author's Disclaimer Note: This book is based on actual events,
but dates may not be accurate. Some of the characters in the story
have fictitious names and some don't, and I have eliminated or
altered details in some cases to protect the person's identity.

This book was published by BookCrafters, Parker, Colorado.
www.bookcrafters.net
bookcrafterscolorado@gmail.com

This book may be ordered from
Amazon.com
and other online bookstores.

Dedicated to
the Forgotten Survivors
of Traumatic Brain Injury:
The Families

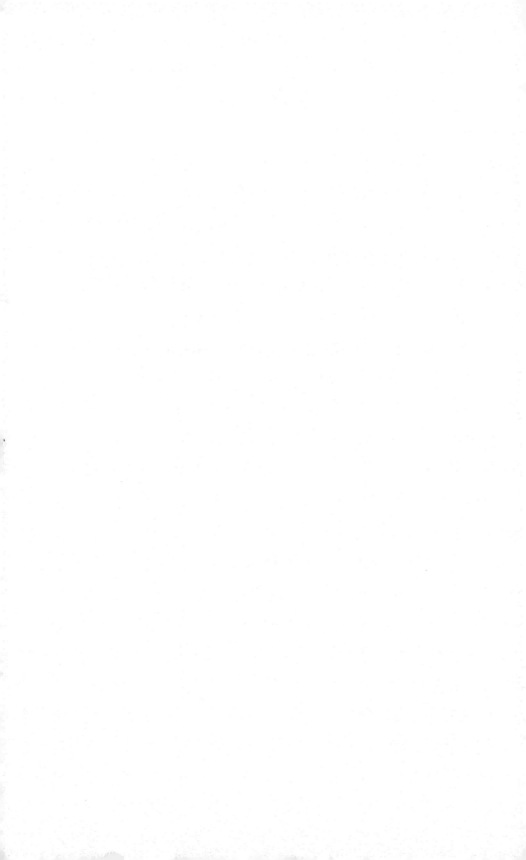

I wish this book could be available to all families after the initial shock of suffering a TBI wears off. I have felt every one of the emotions Janis so eloquently expressed in her book. Families are the "forgotten ones" when a loved one suffers a TBI. They need to see that there is hope and support even though the struggle ahead of them seems overwhelming. Thank you, Janis, for bringing families into the discussion of life after a TBI.

Kim Callahan, Johnstown, CO

No one can predict how the lives of the family of a TBI survivor will forever be changed. In telling her story, Dr. Ruoff has shared her experiences before and after her son, Jeff's, TBI. Dr. Ruoff's heartbreak led her to find the strength and resolve to cope, and to flourish professionally and personally in a way she could never have imagined prior to Jeff's accident. Jeff provides powerful insights throughout the book about the awakening mind of a TBI survivor. This book should be recommended reading for every family experiencing the pain of living with a loved one with traumatic brain injury. The military should hand them out to all TBI survivors' families!

Betsy Cromwell, Alexandria, VA

Table of Contents

Section III

Introduction

*"General Secretary Gorbachev, if you seek peace,
if you seek prosperity for the Soviet Union and
Eastern Europe, if you seek liberalization: Come
here to this gate! Mr. Gorbachev, open this gate!
Mr. Gorbachev, tear down this wall!"*

—President Ronald Reagan
Brandenburg Gate West Berlin, Germany
June 12, 1987

TIME MAGAZINE DID A SPECIAL ISSUE on the year 1989, calling it "The Year That Defined Today's World." Even though I don't think they had me in mind when the editors decided to do that publication, it was the year that redefined my world. My son Jeff's car crash in 1989, and his traumatic brain injury (TBI), changed him forever and was a catalyst for me chipping away at the walls of my life to become the person I am today, someone I never knew I could be. As I read that issue of *Time*, I was overwhelmed by the significance of that year for the world and our family. The ripple effects of Jeff's TBI transformed our entire family just as the effects of certain events in the world changed the way nations relate to each other.

When the Berlin Wall came down in 1989, two years after Ronald Reagan's impassioned speech in Berlin, I heard about it and reflected back to the year 1974 when my husband, Steve, was stationed in

Frankfurt, West Germany as an Army officer. After we had lived there a year we took the kids on a trip to Berlin through East Germany on a train that only traveled at night through what was the Soviet Union's post World War II territory, stopping at one point for an inspection by East German soldiers along the way. I remembered the next day we were standing in front of the Berlin Wall on the West Berlin side, at the gate called Checkpoint Charlie, looking at the drab greyness of the East Berlin sector on the other side of the wall. I had one year old baby Travis on my hip and a three-year-old Jeff next to me holding my hand, and for the first time I saw why we needed an army as I gazed upward and met the eyes of one of the armed guards standing on the wall with submachine guns pointed directly at us. I had never experienced anything like that before and felt the presence of a powerful, dangerous government; I was sheltered from that in my naive life as an American. It gave me a new appreciation for our safer and freer way of life in the United States. Even though West Berlin was the "free" side of the city it struck me as a kind of metaphor for my life because it was surrounded by the Soviet controlled part of Germany, with the result being that the so-called free West Berlin was actually the walled in part of the city and not East Berlin on the other side of the wall. It was how I had always felt, that the free part of me was trapped in the midst of a life that I felt was oppressive and controlling.

In the seventies no one expected, if they even thought about it, that the Berlin Wall would come down and when it did, in 1989, I was too involved with our family crisis to pay much attention. Things I barely heard about in the news had far-reaching effects on our world, just as the day of February 17, 1989 would have lifelong effects on my life. But when your child is seriously injured nothing else matters and so world events were nothing but a backdrop to me, a blur of newscasts that I heard through muffled ears and saw on the television through eyes clouded by tears. We were just one small family going through our own little drama.

In the same way that I was oblivious to what was happening in Germany, I did not know anything about a genius named Tim Berners-Lee who created the beginnings of the World Wide Web in 1989. That was going to be a very real part of my life someday but at the time I did not know it. The explosion of new technology and social media has led to advancements that help all people with disabilities, but has especially added to the quality of life for so many who face social isolation due to TBI. And for me personally and professionally, the Internet has been a valuable tool for making change when I was lost and confused about direction in my life.

In 1989, the search for freedom and self-expression was a theme in my life. It was something I had valued and fought for in a myriad of ways including separating from my husband and going against the grain of how I was raised to get my advanced education and become, I hoped, a leader in the field of education and disabilities. I had just turned forty and, like many people approaching middle age, I realized I needed to work on figuring out who I was. I had always been a helper but felt that part of me was exhausted. I had always been a rebel who was perhaps too cautious to fully express that side of myself, so I did it on behalf of others.

As the world witnessed the tragic murders in China's Tiananmen Square, when ordinary people rebelled against the oppressive government and lobbied for free speech, I related to it on a personal level. I applauded their brave fight against injustices in the world. This fighting spirit was one of the pieces of my identity I felt I could be proud of, and I was thrilled later to hear that the tyranny exposed by Tiananmen Square led to other countries taking a stand against oppressive governments.

Even though I had been involved with people with disabilities my whole life, and a crusader for their rights, I was naïve in ways I did not even realize. In 1989, before Jeff's TBI, I thought I knew all about the effects of a brain injury from my years of working as a speech-language pathologist, but I was about to find out that I did not understand it at all. And I knew nothing of a new brain injury advocacy movement and had not yet met the leaders of the small but growing National Head Injury Foundation (NHIF) that began in Massachusetts and later moved to Washington DC.

One of the spokespersons and leaders of the NHIF was President Reagan's former Press Secretary James Brady, who would become a part of my life and someone Jeff and I would both come to know. James Brady and the traumatic brain injury he lived through when he was shot in the head during the attempted assassination on the President in 1983 was only a sad story on the television to me at the time. But ten years later, because of what happened to my son, I got the opportunity to know him as a wonderful person and amazing advocate for gun control and people with brain injuries. He always remembered me and asked "How's Jeff?" whenever I saw him, and I was honored to have him as a guest lecturer in my classes after I became a professor teaching courses on brain injury.

1989 was a time of great change around the world and was the year that we saw the Cold War, something I had grown up with, beginning to end as people of numerous countries were speaking out. People who previously were disconnected from each other began to envision a world of globalization and seamless communications among countries and states. It was a profound time and the beginning of enormous change.

But this is not a book about world history; it is about one ordinary family's history and the way that unplanned events transformed our life and pushed me to become a different person able to live without the barriers I put up around me. Like the divided city of Berlin, I had my own armed guards in my head, and I had accepted a lot of propaganda in my life that kept me walled in. I was not happy and it took completely unpredictable life circumstances for me to see that the oppressive force in my life was me.

Walls keep us trapped but they also protect us, and I was afraid. It took a lot of trauma for me to crash through mine and get to a place of inner freedom where I could begin having a new and better life. In recent years I have come to believe that there are two kinds of people in the world; there are those who live their lives based on fear and self-doubt, and there are those who don't have fears (or if they do they just don't pay attention to them). Before 1989 I led a fear-based life, afraid of expressing myself, and that kept me from doing the things I wanted to and knew I needed to do. I believe I'm a different person now and for that I'm grateful.

I have spent twenty-seven years going back-and-forth between obsessing over 1989 and trying to forget those painful times in my life. I have told my story, our family's story, in bits and pieces to audiences when I did presentations or taught classes on brain injury, but there is so much I couldn't talk about or was afraid to. Finally, I am doing what people kept telling me to do, and what my inner voice said I needed to do, which was: write that book. This is that book, the book I have been avoiding, had sleepless nights over, the one I can't bring myself to release into a world of people I don't know and potential critics. You'll notice that I chose to tell the story of 1989 itself in the present tense, although the events themselves are long past. That's because it's a year that never fades from memory, a year imprinted on my brain as if it is all still happening. It's almost too personal to write, and yet that is what I hope will speak to someone who reads it and who might be going through a similar difficult time.

I invite readers to see our story as just one example of the millions of families affected every year by traumatic brain injury or other tragedy, and I hope that our story will promote new understanding about the effects of TBI. I also would like to think that our family's journey will help someone to believe that life can go on and even improve afterward. Because of the many veterans affected by TBI and Post Traumatic Stress Disorder (PTSD), and new publicity about sports injuries and concussion, and the terrible effects of repeated injuries to the brain, there is increased awareness of the need for research and programs to help people with brain injuries.

But I worry that the overlooked puzzle piece—one that has always been missing in the work on the problems of TBI—is the long-lasting repercussions on the family system.

TBI is not a medical event; it is not over when the medical crisis and interventions end. A TBI brings dramatic changes in the person affected that will alter the survivor's life and that of those around the survivor, possibly forever. It is a catalyst for enormous changes, for everyone, though the results will be different for each person or family.

I would love to hear from readers about your reactions after reading what I have written. You may send me a note using the email address of: Ruoffpubandtrng@gmail.com.

Section I

I don't remember much about that time but I know that on February 17, 1989 my life felt chaotic. High school would be over soon and adult life would begin. My parents were separated and I had the social crises common to late adolescence which, of course, felt like major life issues to me. All of this propelled me to crash head-on into a carpet company's van that was on delivery. Aside from the birth of my child and, of course, my own birth, no other events have had such a significant impact on my life.

—Jeff Bouck, TBI Survivor

Chapter 1

Saving Jeff
1989

FUTURISTS, PEOPLE WHO STUDY current trends and use them to predict the future, say we each have multiple futures and I believe that is true. We start life with all sorts of possibilities, and at any moment we can change the path we are on. Which of the many possible futures we get depends on the choices we make amid unforeseen circumstances. Every time I get comfortable and think I know what my life is all about, something changes and I find out I have no control over anything.

Although I know I may sound crazy saying this, and I am not even sure it's real, I have had experiences that may indicate I have some intuitive ability to foresee future events before they happen. One time when I was pregnant, in 1971, I had a dream about my brother getting married to a woman who, so far as I knew, he had never met and I did not know. I told my mother and we laughed about it because my brother did not date much, but she said he had told her earlier that morning that he had a date with someone new the night before and he really liked her and, coincidentally, she did have the same name I told her from my dream. Two years later that person I dreamt about was his wife. A little over a year ago I was driving home from work about a half mile from the house, on our street, and I had to stop because I could not see. I was blinded by a sea of blood red spilling across the road and covering the windshield of my car. I arrived home shaking and terrified and I told my husband, Steve, I thought someone was going to have a horrible car accident on our street. I was afraid it would be my son Jeff, but knew I had unreasonable fears of car accidents from things that happened in my childhood. I pushed the experience to the place in my mind where I put all of my secret ideas and fears, but I still wonder what it means.

My weekdays usually begin with waiting until my two teenage sons, Jeff and Travis, are on the school bus to go to work. But sometimes I have to take them if they miss the bus and then I'm late getting from the Maryland suburbs where we live to my office at Gallaudet University in the heart of Washington DC. I am an Assistant to the Dean of the School of Education and Human Development at Gallaudet and I'm also working toward a Ph.D. although I don't know what my dissertation topic will be or if I will ever finish.

Gallaudet's a special place to me but I'm aware that my friends and family don't always understand that because I'm not Deaf and it's known as the university for Deaf people. It's a university with a heart, an ideal place for crusaders like me. I saw this right away when I first walked into the Department Chair's office to apply for the doctoral program. He had Man from La Mancha (Don Quixote), by Miguel de Cervantes, on his office wall, the exact same print that I have in our living room. I knew I had found what I was looking for; a place where I belonged.

And I've learned so much from my Deaf professors and friends there. It's worth the effort to learn sign language, make sacrifices to take classes and work, and spend the extra time commuting. I don't enjoy the drive some days because the traffic is so bad that even screaming ambulances can't get through. At those times I wonder:

what if someone was in there dying? People can be so indifferent to the suffering of others and I hate that part of human nature.

Last year I was involved in a big Deaf rights movement at Gallaudet called Deaf President Now, or DPN, and helped to fight for the first Deaf President of a University that should be promoting leadership of Deaf people anyway. We held rallies that were televised nationally, and we marched on the Capitol. I did my part as a hearing person by collecting linens from local linen supply companies to be used for banners, and I got the experience of listening to some of the business owners tell me their stories about marching with Dr. Martin Luther King, Jr. in the sixties. They were supportive of the efforts the Deaf community and Gallaudet were making on behalf of Deaf people everywhere. I'm proud of that and of my work at the university, and when I'm on campus I feel important. I'm part of the student leadership and President of the campus honor society, but at home my marriage is a mess and the kids pretty much ignore me unless I'm cooking for them or driving them where they want to go.

I am the only female in this family and I resent that what's important to me doesn't matter to anyone else. Sometimes Steve, Jeff, and Travis all stare at me like I'm speaking a foreign language and then go back to talking about cars or electronics or something I find boring like how to use a particular kind of tool in the garage.

I have to work at getting involved in conversations in my own home. Like when I was caught up in the emotional momentum of DPN and I called the Grease Man, a popular and controversial radio host, and told him what was going on. The Gallaudet protests were a big story on the news around the country and my Deaf friends asked me, as a hearing and speaking person, to help get the word out on the radio. The Grease Man even put me on the air and did one of his weird songs about what I said! When I told the boys at dinner that night, Travis, who was fourteen at the time, immediately went from only half paying attention to a look of teenage horror.

"Mom, you called the Grease Man?" He glared at me and Jeff laughed. Jeff enjoys seeing Travis and I argue for some reason.

"I just hope my friends didn't hear you!" Travis said. It was all about him of course.

I love my family but life at home has been so distressing for years that I don't want to be there. Steve and I have been separated off and on for the past three years and sometimes I get lost in depression and frustration because I don't know what to do; I'm not happy the way things are but I can't seem to change it. I enjoy the weekends to catch up around the house or spend time with my kids and friends, but the future is so uncertain that much of the time I don't really enjoy anything. I just smile and try to keep up pretenses of being happy, something I'm good at as I'm discovering. When Steve is living with me I am mad at him, when we are apart I miss him and want to work on our marriage, and at the times I am convinced we are heading for divorce all I want to do is go out and experiment with meeting other men. I feel like I'm as much of a teenager as my kids are and that I should feel guilty for how I'm acting, but the truth is I don't feel guilty at all and that's what I feel the most guilt about. I want to be happy and have a stable family life but it seems that it isn't possible to have both, at least not with Steve.

On a cold Saturday afternoon Jeff and I sit at a McDonalds near our house and talk about the ironic overlap of our lives with both of us, mother and teenage son, out there in the dating scene. I think this is one of the oddest things about being a single parent of two boys and I ask him, "What if we ran into each other out somewhere?" I laugh and he looks disturbed, as if that possibility had not occurred to him before. I am enjoying this conversation.

"I just thought of something really funny," I say. "I have a date this weekend with that guy named Jerry, who you have met, and I think he's in his late fifties. And the other day I had a coffee date with someone else named Jason who is almost the same age as you. He wants me to go out with him sometime."

He stares at me bug-eyed. "Wait. What? How old is this guy?"

I try not to laugh. "He's twenty-four but when we met I thought he was about thirty, closer to my age, and he apparently thought I was just a few years older than him. Don't worry; I don't think I want to go out with him anymore."

I am feeling rather cool that I look young enough to do something like that, and I like to shock my sons once in a while and remind them I'm not just their mom.

"He's a bondsman," I add to complete the zinger. "I've never dated a bondsman before!"

"Mom, you need to stay away from him," he says in a serious, parental tone. "I mean it. I know guys like him and they're trouble."

"Okay, I won't go out with him," I say, still chuckling.

I enjoy talking to Jeff and always have. We move on from the uncomfortable topic of dating to other subjects like what's going on at school and my new car that he wants to drive.

Jeff will be eighteen soon and I know there are parts of his life he doesn't tell me about, but at least he talks to me. His younger brother, Travis, is a more reserved personality and not interested in hearing about my feelings or discussing his own. I know it's his age, and that he's had Steve for a role model, but sometimes it frustrates me because my kids are my family, the most important part of my life. I want us to have the connection I don't have with my husband and never did.

"You just spill your feelings all over the place," Travis told me once when I was driving them to school. "I don't like it."

I sighed through my tears, but at least he's honest.

Jeff laughed and said, "I like it Mom, so you can tell me. Having feelings is quite logical you know."

It's not that Travis and I have a bad relationship. When he was little he was the cuddly one who said he wanted to marry me. And even though he keeps me at a distance now we do talk, but we do best when it's about things like what's for dinner, can he go to the movies with his friends, current events in the news, or decisions that need to be made around the house, stuff like that.

With Steve gone I rely on Travis for some of the handyman jobs around the house, things his dad used to do, because he's good at fixing anything and enjoys it. Travis and I discuss literally the nuts and bolts of life more than anything touchy-feely like relationships. My psychiatrist, Dr. Stone, has told me I would do better with him if I stayed out of his head so I'm trying to do that. I think in general I have a good relationship with both of my sons and we function well as a three-person single parent family unit, probably because we've had lots of practice even before Steve and I separated. From the time they were babies there were too many times that Steve was not with us because of being in the Army. I have a lot of resentment and feelings of abandonment that I know have contributed to me wanting out of the marriage. But Steve and I always try to put our differences aside for family holidays and special occasions, and I'm glad we can do that.

On February 1, 1989 we take the boys out to dinner at one of our favorite local restaurants called the Olney Ale House, to celebrate Jeff's eighteenth birthday. I can't wrap my brain around the fact that Jeff is old enough to legally move out, go to college, join the military, or do whatever he wants to with the next phase of his life. Travis will be right behind him too and then what? I'll be alone if Steve and I can't work things out. My father said, in one of his nasty letters to me a few months ago, that I have traded my family for a Ph.D. and will be a lonely old lady who no one will want to be with. He has always liked to predict doom and gloom for me so I try to ignore it but it's in my head and I can't get rid of it. I don't read his mail or answer his calls anymore because of that. In fact, I've developed a mailbox phobia because I never know when he or my mother will send me an upsetting letter. I worry that my relationship with men will always be troubled because of him too. So I am afraid to let go of Steve because he has been the one man I have always been able to count on, at least until now, even though I have known for a long time we are not right for each other.

Steve and I have a deeply flawed and complicated relationship. We've been moving in and out of each other's lives for years, saying we still love each other and yet doing irreparable harm to one another and our marriage. I hate Steve at times, maybe because he is who he told me he was when we were young and I just didn't accept it. And I hate him because I am afraid I will always love him and I don't want to. He doesn't want to solve our problems; he just wants me to go back to being the same person I was when we met and I can't do that. I'm twenty-four years older and I'm too hurt by his indifference to my wants and needs, and I'm aware now of the way he never asks me how I feel about anything.

I think the biggest problem I have, one I don't like admitting, is that I'm scared that my father is right. I feel like I'll die without people to live with, take care of, depend on, and to call my family. I am trying my best to adjust to a new life without my husband, if that happens, but secretly I am still hopeful that our family will get through this rough patch and be restored to normal, even to a new and improved version. I have an old romanticized idea that Steve and I will develop a different kind of relationship that is not the same as what we had as teenagers.

"How do you know you love me?" I asked Steve in 1966 as we were making out to Johnny Mathis songs in my parents living room. He smiled at me.

"Because I want to take care of you," he said.

That was it; I was a goner. I always called him my Knight in Shining Armor and he loved that reflection of him in my eyes.

"I'm not who you think I am," he told me once when we were about to graduate from high school. "I'm not really a nice person. I don't care about anyone but myself."

I remember that I argued with him because I thought that I knew him better than he did. Why do we women do that? I'm learning that men do tell you who they are and I should listen. The guy who says "I'm not good at commitment" isn't going to be with just me, and the one who says "I'm not very honest" is going to lie. I need to accept how Steve really is but I don't want to; I still want to change him and us and I keep going back to a belief that maybe, if I try harder, things will get better, who knows.

The other problem I have with Steve is that I can't stay away from him and every time we are together we end up making love. It feels like he is a drug I'm addicted to rather than a husband, like the way I can't stop binging on junk food when I'm upset or drinking too much at parties. Does that make me an addict? I worry that I am an alcoholic like my father and a few other family members, but I can't think about that because I am overwhelmed with just trying to put my marriage back together.

We all have a good time as a family celebrating Jeff's eighteenth birthday and I feel close to Steve because we are parents together and our kids are important to both of us. He stays with me overnight and I am confused again. I know we still love each other. We can work this all out; I know we can.

A few days later I call Steve's apartment on Saturday morning and a woman answers his phone in a sleepy voice.

"I'm sorry, I must have the wrong number," I say.

"Are you looking for Steve?" she asks. I am confused so I hang up, my heart racing in panic.

Steve calls me back right away.

"Janis," he says. "I didn't want you to find out this way."

Find out what? My head is spinning and I feel nauseated. He told me he was not dating anyone, he still says he loves me, so what is it exactly that I am finding out?

I barely hear him as he begins to explain that she works in his office, is just a friend, and she's using his apartment as a place for her and her children to crash while she separates from her cheating husband.

I want to believe him, like I always wanted to believe him when he said he would get out of the Army but never did. Or when he told me over and over he was two, three, or six hours late because he was helping someone in distress. And when the bill collectors called and he explained that they just had their information wrong.

My kids tell me they have known about this woman, Cynthia, for a couple of years. How is it that I had no idea?

I'm back on the roller coaster. It feels like life is once again spinning out of control and I am not in the driver's seat at all. Travis is the one I can count on to tell me the truth and not spare my feelings so I ask him questions until he gets tired of being the informant and says that's all he knows.

"Mom, give it up," he says. "Just get a divorce."

I value his opinion but don't want to accept that it's over with Steve. It's crazy because I'm the one who wanted out, the one who thought for years that I never should have married Steve in the first place, and yet I'm hanging on. I know I have problems with accepting my problems. Dr. Stone says my problems are different than I think they are, but I don't know what to do with that. Steve has always told me I just expect too much and that I need to be happy with what I have. But I've tried and it doesn't work. So Travis is probably right.

I want to think my marriage and my kids are just fine even when the evidence tells me otherwise. My brother, a lawyer, always told me I'd probably be a better lawyer than him, but I know that's not true because I don't trust my own perceptions about anything. I'm at a point now where I'm questioning everything in my life. Have I been asleep at the wheel all these years? How is it that I never saw Steve as a cheater and a liar, just as a nice guy, if a little boring, who was often in the wrong place at the wrong time? He never trusted me and I bought it; I believed I was a flake and the one who was not loyal and consistent. What else have I been misreading? I'm afraid that my whole life has been a lie and that terrifies me.

Travis also told me recently that Jeff is speeding when he drives, and I know Travis never says things like that unless it is important. He and Jeff have the "brother's code" as they call it. They don't rat on each other. They cover up for each other when they sneak out at night, and they don't tell each other's secrets, especially to me. When I question Jeff about his alleged speeding he laughs at me and says he is not speeding all that much. He says Travis exaggerated.

I am worried about Jeff because he's so smart but does some really stupid things. He has a very high IQ but was diagnosed with Attention Deficit Disorder (ADD) two years ago, and maybe that explains his behaviors but it seems to me that it's more than that. He gets so depressed and then at other times he acts like he's on top of the world, and that's when he lies to me. I'm starting to see that Jeff is pretty rebellious and out of control, but I have no idea how to handle it.

Whenever I try to talk to Steve about Jeff and his behaviors I get a response like "Oh he'll be fine, he's just like me." I guess that's supposed to make me feel better, but deep inside my stomach turns when he says that. That's a signal I'm beginning to recognize; the little voice inside that says to trust my perceptions. I ignore it though because I don't know what to do with that kind of problem that seems to have no solution. Better to forget about the problem.

Part of me thinks it's good that my sons are strong willed and hard for me to handle at times because it means they think for themselves and are able to grow up and be assertive. Dr. Stone, tells me that I don't need to be both parents, that Steve should be the father and disciplinarian with boys at this age. He says I should just be their mom. We had a discussion about that one day.

"But he can't do it," I say when he tells me Steve should be more firm with the boys.

"But he should," he says.

"But he can't!" I continue to say, and we go back-and-forth like that until I give up. I get the point, that if I don't stop trying to father them Steve never will. And it's not working anyway.

Jeff is old enough that I decide I have to let him make his own bad choices and learn from them. Like the time he and his friends drove to Ocean City one weekend a few months ago. He went without permission and the old Volkswagen Steve's grandparents gave him broke down on the Bay Bridge. I left it up to Steve and Jeff to handle. They did, even though Steve probably didn't tell Jeff he should not have been going to O.C. in the first place.

Steve had to go rescue them and have the car towed, and when he was home Jeff and I argued. That's when I told him, "I give up! Just make your own damn decisions!"

After this phone call, I am thinking that it's no wonder Steve hasn't been very actively involved as a parent; he has another family in the wings of his life. I am in shock, realizing that all of them, my husband and sons, are all living a life I know nothing about. I want to run away; I just can't handle this. I can't deal with a deceitful husband and teenage sons who are rebellious and secretive. I can't sleep. I lay awake every night crying my heart out, feeling sick to my stomach all the time. I don't know what to do and can't picture any future without our family together. I can't trust anyone, not even me.

I am not even excited that the Dean, Dr. Dave Martin, has asked me to represent him at a professional conference on higher education in St. Louis, Missouri. I should be happy that I am going to the conference to meet with people about Deaf education and represent the Dean because it's a wonderful networking opportunity for me. But I don't know how I will be able to present a professional appearance when I am trapped in a tornado of emotions and tears.

On Friday, February 17, I pack a suitcase to leave for the conference. I remind myself this is a huge honor and will help to get me out of the anger that turns quickly to numbness, the feeling that nothing about me or my career matters. Jeff drives me to the Rockville metro station about two miles away and we chat about his life and what they will do while I'm gone for three days. He's happy to have the use of my sporty new Pontiac Corsica, so different from the Volkswagens and Hondas I'd driven previously. Buying that Pontiac was my nod to being forty years old and entitled to the same midlife crisis as any man.

Jeff assures me that after he takes me to the metro he will go on to the high school and then, over the weekend, he and Travis will stay with their dad at his apartment. I am uneasy about them there with this woman I don't know and her two young children. Steve's apartment only has one bedroom and a small den with bunk beds that our kids use; apparently her kids now sleep in those beds so Jeff and Travis have to camp out in the living room. I hate it that he gave our sons' bunk beds to her kids. It's ridiculous, I know, because Jeff is over six feet tall and Travis is close to that. They outgrew those beds long ago, but still it's as if Steve is giving away our kids and replacing them with hers.

On the Metro Red Line I ruminate all the way to Union Station where I catch a city bus for the rest of the trip, and try to convince myself the family upheaval may be a good thing in the long run. Is it really the end of the world if Steve and I do get divorced? I'll be free of trying to make a marriage work that just doesn't. Even the marriage counselor, and now our kids, have all told me to give up. Steve has probably done me a service by forcing me to accept that the marriage is over. How many people need to show me that brick wall before I stop crashing into it?

I know I need to change direction in my life and go around the walls to see what's on the other side. It might be exactly what I want. But Steve and I have been together for so long that I'm afraid I can't ever let go. I don't believe this other relationship he has is real; it can't be. I can't stop myself from wondering how I could change him, or things in our relationship, and make things right with us again.

Once I'm at the office I talk to Dave about the conference and get my plane ticket. Mid-morning a taxi picks me up in front of the university to take me to National Airport and after I check my bags I board a Trans World Airline (TWA) flight, find my seat halfway down the aisle, settle in and fasten my seat belt. I try to relax. I close my eyes, take a deep breath, and think about how good it will be to get away. This may be just what I need to get my head straight.

The Captain announces over the intercom that we will depart in a few minutes, and then a flight attendant appears at the front of the cabin and calls my name. What? I look around wondering if I heard right, and then he says it again. I raise my hand and he makes his way down the aisle to my seat, hunches over to talk low and tells me to follow him. As I fumble with my seatbelt, I ask what this is about. He says "There's been an accident."

I see other passengers staring at me as I grab my purse, and I feel myself beginning to shake. I follow the flight attendant from the plane down the off-ramp and into the airport and it feels like another ten miles to get through the airport to the TWA office. I am led to a chair and handed a phone, and someone gets me a glass of water as I pick up the phone and put it to my ear.

"Hello?" I say still trembling, my heart pounding. I wait and hear only the muffled, unintelligible sounds of background noise on the other end of the phone.

After a few seconds Steve's voice is telling me Jeff has been in a car accident, and he does not know yet if he is dead or alive. He says the police are on another line giving him details as they find out. I have the sense that this is all a bad dream, or a lie, and I will wake up to find myself back on the plane, flying through the clouds to St. Louis and the conference. Then Steve says that the police have confirmed Jeff is alive and has been transported to Suburban Hospital in Bethesda. I am to meet him there.

I feel so lost; I don't know what to do. What about my suitcase? How do I get to the hospital? I can't breathe and can't talk clearly, and all I know is that I have to be at Suburban Hospital right now. I have to get to Jeff but I am worried about my suitcase. It's on the way to Missouri. No, I am told, they took my suitcase off the plane. How did they know to do that? Where is it now?

Someone with the TWA staff leads me to the front of the airport and hails a taxi for me, and he tells me the airline will deliver my bags back to my house later so I don't need to worry about that. I think with curiosity that they must have handled things like this before. I wonder: how often does this happen? My thoughts are random and unfocused as I fight against the river of tears that I hear roaring inside my head ready to burst through the dam.

As I get into the taxi, The TWA representative hands a voucher to the driver and tells him where I am going but the driver doesn't like that. He is arguing in a thick foreign accent about the voucher; he does not want to accept it. He wants cash which I don't have. I start to cry and the TWA representative intervenes and convinces the cabbie to take the voucher. As we drive away from the airport he is still complaining, saying the vouchers are not worth anything because they don't pay him. I yell at him telling him I don't care what he wants because my son is hurt and I need to get to the hospital.

The ride to the hospital around the Washington DC Beltway in late morning traffic is slow. It takes forty-five minutes, maybe an hour, to get there. Tears roll non-stop down my face and I lay my head back against the seat and give in to sobs as the reality sets in. Jeff, oh Jeff; how could this happen to you? I can't stand the images that come into my mind's eye of him trapped in that car, maybe bleeding, hurting, scared, and alone. Oh God, I don't want to lose him.

When I walk into the Emergency Room there are people standing against the walls on the other side of the room watching me and I barely see them through the veil of tears. I try to focus and become aware of the high school principal, the school counselor, and some of Jeff and Travis's friends, and I smile weakly in their direction but I can't talk to them. Travis appears and takes my hand and a nurse guides us to a sofa and begins to explain.

She tells me, "Your son is okay, but he has what we call a closed head injury," as if I have no understanding of what that is. I bristle. I am insulted and I inform her in a disdainful voice that I know what a head injury is because I am a speech-language pathologist, and I know that it is serious and that he is not okay so please don't be so condescending. She smiles and asks if I would like a glass of water.

People talk to me, offering their sympathy and support, but the only person I can let into the protective bubble I am putting around myself is Travis who sits next to me holding my hand and trying to comfort me. After a while Steve appears with another man beside him, a friend of his I don't know but whom Steve has mentioned before. He is a doctor at Walter Reed Army Medical Center where Steve works as a hospital administrator.

Steve is grinning as if he is going to a party and I think he looks psychotic given the circumstances. But he has always done that, acted as if things are okay when they are not. He tells me his friend is a doctor, which I tell him I know, and that he is there to help us understand what has happened. I know the friend is a urologist, so I wonder how that's going to be helpful since urology has little to do with head injuries. I can barely look at Steve because I am so angry at him, and yet I need him and want him there. I remind him that we have to pull together for our family, for Jeff.

I tell the nurse I want to see Jeff, no matter what condition he is in, but she says we have to wait until the doctors finish working on him. I try to explain that I don't care what he looks like; I just need to be with him. He is my child and he is hurt, so I need to be there, but she is firm that I have to wait. I hate her.

After about an hour the others finally leave and our little family, plus Steve's friend, are escorted to another room and told the doctor will talk to us soon and then we can see Jeff. We wait another hour or so and I notice that Steve is not there so I go looking for him.

I find him at a hospital pay phone talking to his girlfriend, and I completely lose my mind.

"No!" I scream and I begin hitting him. "You can't do this!"

I feel the blood rush to my head as I pass out, and then someone, maybe Steve, picks me up and carries me to a small room, like a storage closet, where I am left alone. It's as if there is a different person inside of me who has emerged and I have no control over what I'm doing anymore. I can't stop screaming and crying because my son has been hurt and my husband is talking to his girlfriend and not me, and because the world is an unsafe place. Travis comes in to try to quiet me but I am still hysterical and he leaves in anger. He thinks I am mad at him and he won't listen when I tell him I'm not.

When I finally calm down, exhausted, and come out of the tiny room, Steve tells me he was just calling Cynthia to let her know what happened and to tell her that he is at the hospital and doesn't know when he will be home. So I'm just overreacting? He acts as if I'm crazy to be so upset and tries to hug me but I don't let him. My tears continue like a leaky faucet that drips no matter how hard I try to turn it off. I walk around and talk, and still the tears just flow all by themselves.

We talk to the ER doctor, and I think how tired he looks and what a hard job that must be. "Your son is in a coma," he says, "and we won't know the outcome for at least twenty-four hours. This is a critical period and we just have to wait it out."

He explains about the brain and complicated medical procedures that I don't fully understand and he begins talking to Steve and his doctor friend more than to me. I am angry and I interrupt him.

"I probably know more about head injury than they do," I say. "I'm a speech pathologist, and I would appreciate it if you talk to me and not just to them."

All three of these very tall men stare down at me in surprise and then the doctor apologizes and includes me after that. I begin asking questions and it feels better that at least I can find out something and not have Steve, or his friend who does not belong there, be the point of information.

The ER doctor tells us, "With a traumatic brain injury the first twenty-four hours will determine everything, whether he lives or dies, so he is being carefully monitored. He had a seizure when he was first injured, which is common during a serious head trauma, and he is now on seizure prevention medication."

Seizures? I had not thought of that and I worry about what it means. I have worked with kids who had seizure disorders and I don't want that for Jeff.

There is too much information thrown at us too fast and I try to remember it all but I react to everything I hear with such intense emotions that my own brain feels assaulted. The tired-looking ER doctor says that Jeff has a lot of bleeding and hemorrhaging in his brain and they cannot tell yet where the most extensive damage is. His brain injury is diffuse, spread out all over, rather than limited to a specific part of the brain, and as the brain tissue absorbs the blood they will know more. It's horrifying to picture my son's brain bleeding, absorbing blood and making more blood, shrinking and swelling, doing things that apparently no one can control or predict.

The doctor finally tells us we can go in to see him but warns that Jeff looks pretty bad and we need to be prepared, to which I say we are. But I'm not at all. When I see Jeff lying in that bed my heart is broken. How could any mother, or father, be prepared for the sight of her child lying motionless with tubes inserted into him and bandages covering his head? The expression on his face makes me think he is in horrible pain. I hear him moaning in a low, soft murmur. I tell Travis to go spend the night with his best friend, Jon, and they leave saying they'll be back the next day.

Steve and I stay in the intensive care waiting room that first night, sleeping on chairs we push together to make into a bed, but we sleep only a little because almost every hour there are new reports on the various brain scans done to monitor Jeff's brain as the swelling ebbs and flows like the tide. Some of the bleeding begins to slow down. He is put on oxygen and his natural breathing stopped. I have never heard of this approach and I question the doctor about why it is necessary.

"Does this mean he can't breathe on his own?" I ask the doctor. I'm frightened that he has to rely on a machine to breathe.

"No," he says. "The goal is to prevent further damage that can occur with Jeff's brain swelling inside the skull." He explains that the skull is like a box that the brain sits in, cushioned by fluid; the skull forms the walls of that box. Swelling can further damage the brain tissue that is pressed against the bony ridges inside the skull. If that happens, doctors will have to do surgery to drain the blood and other fluid from Jeff's brain to prevent further damage. The oxygen will shrink the brain and guard against this nightmare scenario. I realize I have to accept the need for Jeff to be hyper-oxygenated and put on a ventilator, but I don't like it.

It's a long night and hard to get any sleep. When we are not listening to medical reports, Steve and I argue, going over old, unresolved issues. We argue because I am doing everything I can to convince him to forget about our problems and put the kids first. Jeff will need all the family support he can get if he makes it through this.

"You don't love her, I know that," I say. "We need to stop our fighting and put our family back together." I tell him I will stop dating and we will go back to marriage counseling and make this right. None of those problems that seemed so important matter to me now; what matters is only our family. Jeff and Travis need us to be a family I tell him.

We eat breakfast in the hospital cafeteria, and when we return to the Critical Care Unit the nurse tell us that Jeff has survived that critical first twenty-four hours and that's good news; they think he will live. All day Saturday we camp out in the waiting room talking to the doctors and nurses and a few friends and neighbors who stop by to wish us well.

Steve's sister shows up with her two kids and they go in to see Jeff. I'm worried about how this will affect them but our nephew, who is eleven years old, comes back and says, "He looks fine to me." I can't help but laugh that he sees Jeff in that condition and thinks he's fine. We see what we want to see and he's a child so I don't say anything.

In the late morning Travis joins us and tells us about a dream he had. He says he dreamed that Jeff came to Jon's bedroom window and knocked on it to wake them up. Travis tells us that in the dream Jeff laughed and said, "Psych! It was all a joke!"

"I wish it was a joke," I say and he looks away. I know Travis, like all of the kids, just wants to believe Jeff will be okay. I do too. It's too hard for any of us to accept what has happened.

When I am half awake and half asleep on the sofa, the waiting room phone rings and Steve's sister answers it.

"No, she's too tired to talk but I'll give her the message," she tells the caller without even asking me what I want. I'm angry with her for that, but I don't have the energy to argue and I know she means well.

Late in the afternoon Steve leaves the hospital to get some of his things from his apartment, and he's gone for a long time. He returns looking drained and tells us that his girlfriend left him a suicide note and disappeared, and he had gone to find her. That's what took so long he says.

"Don't you see how selfish she is?" I ask him with an I-told-you-so tone. He says yes, and he is finished with her. He says he will tell Cynthia she has to move out.

I have kept a diary or journal since I was ten years old and I try to write something every few days, or at least once a week, to keep track of how I'm feeling and what is happening in my life in case I need to remember and can't. At some point, a few years ago, I began writing mostly my dreams to analyze because I was feeling so confused about my past, what I wanted in life, and how I felt about my marriage. I talked endlessly about my dreams in therapy.

But usually I do write some day-to-day things about what's going on in my life.

For the first few days after Jeff's accident, however, I am too upset to write anything in my journal, and too busy going back-and-forth to the hospital.

Five days later, on February 22, I write:

> *On Friday Jeff, my baby, had a head-on collision with a van and now he lies there in a coma, tubes coming out of him, a machine breathing for him, his poor head all damaged and his knee cap shattered. As he improves a little each day my hopes do grow for a full recovery, but inside I am so terrified. I want to grab him up, hold him close, and take him back in time. I want to take everyone, Jeff, Travis, Steve and me and go somewhere safe. Steve went to his apartment to get things and to end his relationship with Cynthia but said he's worried she will try to kill herself again. Later I called his apartment when he wasn't back by 2 a.m. and Cynthia answered. She said Steve was at the hospital and didn't seem to know he was back with me.*

I am able to recall what I believe to be the experience of "waking up" from my coma twenty-six years ago. It seemed to me that I was descending from clouds and was suddenly "there" in my body. To me this memory feels like the earliest memory of my life. I was eighteen years old. To say that my life began at a hospital does not quite describe what I mean. Perhaps it is better to say that my SECOND life began at a hospital.

—Jeff Bouck, TBI Survivor

Chapter 2

Jeff Is an Interesting Referral

WE ARE WAITING. When your child is hurt like this, in a life or death situation, nothing else matters; time stops and the rest of the world floats by in suspended animation as you wait to find out what will happen. You remember so much like how he was born after a long and difficult labor during a dust storm in El Paso, Texas and that he had a skull fracture from induced labor, and how you had to put him in the window after you took him home because he was jaundiced and needed the sunlight. You smell his new baby breath and remember how surprisingly sweet it was, and you hear his infant cries from the bassinet beside your bed. You think about his big blue eyes and how smart he was when he was only seven months old and saying his first words: ma-ma, da-da, shoe, and "Maah!" which meant our dog, Max. You remember the way he would lie on his tummy when he was five months old, and how he would cry in frustration when he tried to push himself up and scoot but couldn't quite do it. You can still hear his baby voice when he was eight months old and would go from room to room in his walker looking for you when you played hide and seek, calling out "Ma-ma!" You think about those special times like when he was in first grade and all on his own he got the school bus driver, who had a framing shop, to frame your favorite picture of him and his baby brother and give it to you for a surprise present at Christmas.

While you wait helplessly you watch that child go from being an active, strong, fiercely independent, intelligent, and healthy young man to being a comatose patient, a case in a medical file. Whatever other problems you have, like your husband living with his secretary, don't matter anymore. What matters is a lot of technical jargon and medical procedures that you want to object to but can't, and your child's struggle to stay alive. You pray whether you believe in God or not.

I look at Jeff's medical records on February 24, 1989 and read:

"Jeffrey Bouck is an 18-year-old male who was involved in a head-on motor vehicle accident on February 17, 1989. He was brought to Suburban Hospital unconscious but moving all extremities, right side greater than left. A seizure was witnessed with subsequent initiation of anticonvulsant medication. He was also immediately intubated and hyperventilated. CT scan of the head has shown bifrontal contusions with a small right subdural hematoma producing a very mild right to left shift. Follow-up CT scan within the last day or two has shown partial resolution of these bleeds. Additional injuries have included a right patellar fracture which was openly reduced and internally fixated on February 21, 1989. Current medications include Decadron, Zantac, Dilantin, phenobarbital, Carafate, Nafcillin, Gentamicin, and Rocephin. His clinical course has been complicated by pneumonia."

The report describes the clinical examination and goes on to say:

"Mr. Bouck is recovering from a severe closed head injury as well as a fractured right patella. Although he remains unresponsive to verbal commands, he has apparently shown lightening of his coma over the last two to three days."

The doctor requests physical and occupational therapy consults as well as daily bedside therapy for Jeff. He adds:

"As soon as he is off the ventilator, then remobilization can become more aggressive. The prognosis is guarded at this time. Thank you for this interesting referral."

My son has become not only a patient in a coma but also an interesting referral with a guarded prognosis. What does that mean, what is guarded about his chance for recovery? There are so many questions and they stick in my throat like peanut butter that I sometimes eat by gobs when I don't know how to cope with life and the hunger I feel for something, anything that will soothe me and make the pain go away.

I feel like both Jeff and I have been invaded. He lies in a bed loosely covered by a sheet—he is naked to let wounds heal—with tubes coming out of him and an artificial machine breathing for him. I can't accept this; I won't.

During the first week after Jeff's accident Steve and I spend every day by Jeff's bedside. Then Steve says he has to go back to work and will be at the hospital in the evenings and on weekends. I am alone each day with Jeff and my thoughts and fears. My new car has been totaled in the accident, and I don't have a rental car yet, so Steve drops me off at the hospital in the morning. I can't go home until Steve or someone else picks me up in the evening, but that's fine with me because there is nowhere else I want to be anyway. I would move into Jeff's hospital room if they would let me.

I do have another child though and I am worried about him and about how little time or energy I have for Travis. I know he is a resourceful fifteen, almost sixteen-year-old but he is on his own too much, getting rides or taking the bus to the hospital after school every day unless he has something else he has to do. There are times I don't know what he's doing. Sometimes he is with his friends and I know they are at our house unsupervised, but I can't do anything about it. I want Steve to be there and to be a firm father to Travis but he isn't, or can't, or won't and I can't do anything about that. In fact, right now, I don't feel like I have any control over any part of my life. I have never felt so alone and afraid.

I need people to help but I don't know who I would ask or what I would ask for, and I don't believe anyone could understand the deep and profound anguish I carry inside all of the time anyway. I've never been good at telling people when I'm hurting and this is the very worst kind of hurt so, no, I do not want to talk about it. I just want this to be over with. I especially hate it when people tell me we are "so lucky" Jeff is alive. How is any of this lucky? How can people say things like that? I know they mean well but it feels dismissive and cruel like the way my family always dismissed my feelings as a child.

Steve called my parents the day after Jeff's accident to tell them what had happened and they said that they would fly to Maryland and plan Jeff's funeral. I guess to them he's already dead? My sons are their only grandchildren and I want support from them that I know I will never get so I don't even let myself think about it except that I can't help but think of it; I have friends who I know do have families that would help them when they have problems. I've begun to realize, however, that my parents never make me feel better when things go wrong in my life; they just point out all of my faults and how I need to change who I am. Right now I can't handle that.

I started therapy two years ago after years of running away from my fears and depression, and right now I'm so grateful to have my standing appointments with Dr. Stone, even though there are days I show up and spend the entire fifty minutes doing nothing but crying and saying things like, "Jeff doesn't deserve this; this can't be happening to him!" Sometimes I feel like I'm going to levitate from the couch because I'm in so much emotional pain I just roll around holding my stomach and sobbing.

The process of psychotherapy is always hard, but Dr. Stone is wonderful. I don't know how old he is, and he wouldn't tell me if I asked, but I like to pretend he's a lot older than me so he can be like the father I wish I'd had. He just listens and verifies that what had happened in my life, and what has happened now to Jeff, actually is as awful as it feels; that I'm not imagining things or exaggerating like my parents always tell me.

Loneliness and anger threaten to consume me, and I hate it that all I know to do in retaliation is to consume too much food. It's a problem I've had my whole life but right now I don't know what else to do. Last night I ate pizza with Travis and then devoured an entire frozen cheesecake in front of a TV show I wasn't even watching.

There have been friends and neighbors calling or visiting, but I'm not able to tell any of them how I feel. My two best friends have not been to the hospital and I assume it's because they have kids and this is a parent's worst nightmare. So I just go through the days, sleeping only a little at night. I now live at the hospital trauma ward.

We haven't even met the hospital social worker yet but she left her card and some brochures and pamphlets about TBI and I read them while I sit by Jeff's bed. I try to focus on every detail because I want to understand what has happened. They, whoever wrote these things, say that you should act as if the person in a coma can hear you even if you don't think he can and it's important to talk about things going on in the world. So I do that. I miss Jeff so much I can hardly breathe and it helps to tell him my feelings while I'm with him, except for the big one. I know I can't tell him my fear that he might die. I hope he hears me but I have no idea what is going on with him and what his damaged brain in doing in there trapped behind closed eyes and walled in inside the box called a skull.

"Jeff, I miss you so much and I need you to wake up," I say. I ramble on and on, talking to him like I did when he was little and could not understand everything I was saying but I knew he just enjoyed the feeling of conversation.

"Hey, guess what? Your friends made you a mixed tape with all your favorite songs and groups like Guns N' Roses, Depeche Mode, and The Clash. They said they are bringing them over later!"

Or I say fake cheerful things like "Hi Jeff, it's Tuesday and you would be at school if you were not here in this hospital. I think your friends and teachers will be glad to see you when you get back. Travis even misses you and oh yeah, he's dating a different girl now, but I can't remember her name." I pretend he is laughing with me about that because he would if he could.

The rest of my life is on hold. The world outside of the hospital has become non-existent to me, and I have not been in to work at all nor do I even think about it. I called the Dean's office at Gallaudet the day Jeff was admitted, to let them know I did not go to the conference, and Dave told me to do what I needed for Jeff and to keep them posted on his progress. He knows my kids and has become a wonderful friend as well as my mentor and boss. It's reassuring to know that my Gallaudet community will be there for me when I go back. But right now work and my Ph.D. program are the farthest things from my mind.

I eat my meals alone in the hospital cafeteria and get candy bars from the vending machines, and at night I go home and eat too much and drink too much wine so I can sleep. Steve is still living with me at our house, but he has started going out in the evenings and sometimes does not show up until midnight or later, or even the next morning. I know he's lying to me and I smell cigarette smoke on him, which is the scent of a stranger because I don't smoke, none of our friends smoke, and he has always been adamantly opposed to people smoking and never did smoke himself. He's seeing her I'm sure, but at this point I don't care.

I mark time by how many days Jeff's been in this damn coma. It's the second week. Jeff has developed medical complications like pneumonia and infections. The nurses tell me it is normal for that to happen to a comatose patient because he is inert and has the various tubes for breathing, urination and fluids, liquid food and medications, which can all cause irritations. It still terrifies me that a machine is breathing for my son and I can't stop obsessing over that. He has begun to run a fever. They did tests to rule out meningitis, and more tests to check for reactions to the many drugs he has been on. I am just so scared for him.

The hardest part is that I don't know how I am supposed to feel. My question is this: what exactly is the proper way to feel after your healthy eighteen-year-old son has a car crash that causes his head to be rapidly thrown back-and-forth, causing brain damage? How should I feel when I hear that his forehead slammed into the rearview mirror of the car and that all of this caused massive bleeding in his brain? I hate that he is unable to move, speak, eat, drink, open his eyes, or be continent of bowel and bladder when he's an eighteen-year-old young man who had so much potential. How is a mother, any mother, supposed to feel knowing that her child's life is in jeopardy and at best forever changed? The future, as everyone tells us, is impossible to predict. I understand because I've told people in the past the same thing when I was part of a rehabilitation team; but now I'm a mother and not a therapist so how is it that I'm supposed to be okay with that? I actually know what I feel and it's rage. But maybe that's not how I'm supposed to feel? After all, people still tell me how lucky I am that he's alive. Should I feel grateful for this?

I read in the pamphlets on TBI that about one-and-one-half million people sustain brain injuries each year. I can't believe this happens so often in the world and people don't notice. I wonder how I never thought about it before, how we all go on with our normal lives, laughing and enjoying conversations, while so many endure the unbearable sorrow of having someone they love in a coma or dying. I feel sorry for myself, our whole family, and everyone else in the world going through this torture of waiting to find out if someone will live or die or return to normal.

I feel like Jeff has died, but he hasn't. He's fighting for his life in there, in that little hospital room. So I felt guilty if I give in to my grief, and fear of losing him forever, because then it's like I am betraying him, giving up on him. I don't want to ever give up on either of my kids or ignore their pain like I feel my parents did with me.

When my babies were born, and I held them for the first time, I whispered a promise to each of them that I would always love them and take care of them no matter what. My mother always told me that when I was born her thought was "here is someone who is mine, all mine, and will always love me." That seems backward to me and Dr. Stone agrees. Parents are supposed to want to take care of their children and expect to love them no matter what, not the other way around. I will love Jeff no matter how brain-damaged he is when he wakes up.

I show up one morning to find that someone, maybe the phantom hospital social worker, left a brochure in the waiting room that says "brain injury counts as a death," and that helps. When I read that I cry and give myself permission to go ahead and grieve as if Jeff has died. I am allowing myself now to have a pity party. I don't want to live in the shadows of avoidance and denial anymore, about anything. I want to live in reality, but reality sucks right now.

Every day I station myself next to his bed, like a guard dog, watching anyone who comes near him. No one I think might be incompetent is going to touch him. It's the second week of Jeff's coma and yesterday a young respiratory therapist was working with his ventilator while I hovered a few inches away monitoring her every move. Probably I made her nervous, but whatever the reason she made a mistake and knocked the IV needle out of his arm. Blood spurted onto the floor and she became flustered as she tried to reinsert the needle.

"Get away from him!" I yelled, running to the doorway to get the nurse on duty.

The poor girl left the room crying and later I heard it was her first day on the job. Today I feel bad for upsetting her, and if I see her I will apologize, but my focus is on Jeff's safety. And I feel like there is no time to be nice now; it's not my priority. This is about saving my son's life.

Even though my friends rarely visit, Jeff and Travis's friends do and they talk to me in that uninhibited way teenagers do when they are nervous. It's great and I enjoy their company maybe even more than I would my adult friends; plus I am slowly learning more of what happened the day of the accident.

Jeff and three of his friends were planning to skip school that day as a senior skip day, and they were all going to the beach for the weekend instead of Steve's apartment as I had thought. It seems Jeff was at our house on that Friday morning, after he took me to the metro, with a girl named Deidra who I knew as the girlfriend of Jeff's friend Aidan, but now I wonder if she and Jeff were together. They packed some things and headed to the high school in separate cars, Jeff in my Corsica and her driving her car. Their plan was to pick up the others and leave for Ocean City.

So what happened was that Jeff and Deidra were racing down our street, a long and winding country road with plenty of twists and turns and blind spots, and poor Deidra saw in her rearview mirror that Jeff and a white van had collided head-on. She raced to the high school, about a half mile from the accident, to get boyfriend Aidan and then they all went to Travis's class to get him. Someone, we think maybe a neighbor, called 911 and when they all arrived back at the scene the kids saw Jeff being loaded into an ambulance.

I feel sad for all of them, especially Travis who was there watching from behind the police barricade as rescue workers put Jeff in the ambulance. He was not allowed to go with his brother in the ambulance. He's angry about that and I don't blame him.

"I told them he was my brother," Travis said when he told me the story. "But I guess they didn't believe me and wouldn't let me go with him."

Travis and all of their friends are facing a harsh reality they should not have to know at this age. I wish I could help them, but all I can manage right now is to be at the hospital for Jeff. I told Travis I love him but he needs to talk to his friends and maybe the school counselor. She's been great and offered to help in any way she can.

Time passes, and I think ironically it's like when you are pregnant and the baby is late, only it's definitely not the same excitement and positive feelings of a new baby coming. I hate waiting. Between being an Army wife and having a husband who was so often gone and late getting home at night, and the mother of teenagers who don't come home when they are supposed to, I have had enough of waiting. It's been two-and-a-half weeks, and I can't take it anymore. One day I sit by Jeff's bed and begin crying, and I throw myself on his bandaged chest.

"Jeff, you have to come back to me!" I tell him as if I have that mother's right to give him orders even if he is in a coma. "I don't think I can go on living if you die!"

Suddenly I feel a hand on my back gently patting me and I realize it's Jeff.

I sit up and stare at him, my crying abruptly stopped by the surprise of what just happened.

"You can hear me, can't you?" I say.

His eyes are still closed but his right hand, loosely tied to the railings to prevent him from pulling out tubes, moves slowly. I watch and see him form a weak fist, bobbing it a little up and down for the sign language word "yes."

I am afraid to believe it. I need to test what I am seeing, so I ask him yes-no questions, like "Do you know your name? Are you awake? Do you know where you are?"

He answers my questions with a signed "yes" even though his eyes remain closed and his lips unmoving.

Jeff is coming back to me just like I told him to! He is coming out of his coma!

I run to the nurses and get one of them to come with me and watch as I ask him more questions. I explain that I work at Gallaudet University and Jeff has been around Deaf people and sign language for years. She says, yes, he is definitely responding.

"I've never had a patient use sign language before," she says with a smile, "but this is good!"

I call people to tell them Jeff is awake and then I go to lunch at the hospital cafeteria, eating quickly so I can get back to Jeff. When I return his eyes are open and he is staring at me as if I am a stranger. His expression scares me because he has the dark brooding look of a demented soul and not my son whose beautiful blue eyes are usually bright with wit and intelligence. As I read in the brain injury literature, the lights are on but no one is home. It's unnerving.

His haunted gaze follows me as I walk around the room and we watch each other. I watch him watch me and my excitement grows because I know this is Jeff becoming aware of his surroundings and visual tracking means his brain is healing. As I talk to him he does not respond but I feel he is listening.

Steve and Travis show up later that afternoon and they are excited that Jeff is awake. We all begin to fantasize that Jeff will come home before too long, continue to recover, go back to school, and life will return to normal. One doctor tells us that Jeff is young and healthy, and that someday this will just be "a bad time in his life" and I want to believe that, so I do. I'm learning in therapy that I'm good at believing what I want to or what others want me to. Sometimes it creates problems for me, but at other times it helps me get through something until I'm ready for the harshness of truth.

As the days pass I arrive at the hospital to find Jeff awake for an hour or so, and then I see him go back into his "gone place," wherever that is. He still does not speak but he does nod once in a while and he continues to use some signs and gestures and to watch people. There is a person in there but it isn't clear yet who that person is.

This sitting by my son's bed all day is so hard because I'm his mother and yet I'm also a therapist, a speech-language pathologist, and I feel like I should be doing more to help Jeff. Why not? I worked in hospitals, rehabilitation centers, and schools for years helping other people recovering from traumatic brain injuries, strokes, and all sorts of brain-related problems and now I am supposed to just sit by Jeff's bed and do nothing? I can't.

The hospital has started to provide bedside physical and occupational therapy but I'm told they have no speech therapy available right now; they are short-staffed. So I decide that I will do that therapy myself and I come up with strategies to stimulate the parts of Jeff's brain involved with speech and language. Steve and Travis are there one day as I get the bedside jar of sponges on a stick, those used to wet the lips of a tube-fed, non-eating patient like Jeff, and I rub a wet sponge and ice around his lips. His eyes light up; he likes it. Then I make sounds that he can see, focusing on simple consonants, and wait for him to copy me.

"Buh, buh, buh," I say slowly, smiling encouragement at him and using a sound that he can both see and hear. I switch from a voiced consonant to the voiceless equivalent. "Puh, puh, puh." When he doesn't copy me I try the one that babies love to imitate: Mmmm, mmmmm, mmmm."

He stares at me in confusion and then it all seems to register at one time as if that part of his brain has been stimulated enough and has popped open. He looks surprised as he begins to make noises. We repeat the sounds in unison one at a time and then I try a few simple one syllable words.

After three weeks of silence, Jeff utters his first post-injury word and it's "Mmmm...mom!" I am in tears.

"He's talking!" Travis says in amazement. He and Steve are our audience and they are all smiles, and I am excited. I feel like a healer, a miracle worker.

Jeff keeps saying "Mom," over and over, as if he's amused by the sound of his voice, and I watch new lights come on in his eyes. It's as if his damaged brain in trying to make sense of what he is doing and can't quite grasp it yet.

I am not sure if he even knows that I am "Mom," but so what? Jeff is talking and I get to watch new parts of his brain waking up. What an incredible experience this TBI recovery thing is. He is coming alive and just hearing him speak gives me a new euphoric feeling of hopefulness. I feel privileged to be a part of my son getting a second chance at life. But he's not the same Jeff who dropped me at the metro stop on the morning of February 17, three weeks ago, and now I am troubled by questions no one can answer about what kind of life he will have. Will he finish high school, drive again, go to parties, go off to college?

I know, from reading more these days about brain injury than I ever did before, that emerging from a coma is something people sometimes describe as being like a butterfly coming out of the cocoon. That's a lovely image but I can't help but think that there is another part of the analogy no one goes to. The part I most worry about.

What if he emerges as more of a moth than a butterfly? I think the cocoons look pretty much the same for both moths and butterflies, and you can't tell which it is until the adult insect emerges. Seeing Jeff emerge from his coma is like watching a cocoon open and wanting to see him as a beautiful butterfly spread its brightly colored wings and fly. I feel giddy after being sad for so long, kind of bipolar in a non-chemical way. I'm up and down emotionally, and I am wondering if that's how my life will be for as long as this takes. I'm on the roller coaster of TBI and I can't get off because I feel that if I do, someone—either Jeff or me—will die.

As the days pass after Jeff's awakening, my happiness hangs entirely on him making progress, and I watch for little signs of his brain healing. He has begun to smile with the weird, lopsided smile of someone with the one-sided paralysis called hemiparesis. His entire left side remains paralyzed but his right side is improving and he's moving his right arm and leg a little. I know this means the left side of his brain, which involves speech and language and controls the right side of the body, is recovering faster than the right hemisphere of his brain. I never knew the brain wakes up from a coma piecemeal like this. There is so much I thought I knew about brain injury that I'm learning I was clueless about.

The nurses have begun to get Jeff out of bed every day, even when he is barely alert, and they put him in a wheelchair with straps around his body to hold him upright so he doesn't slide out. Still, he slips down as far as he can and I wonder if slouching like that feels more normal for his brain. It's comical because sometimes he lists far over to the side and looks up at us with his funny grin, We all laugh but it's a nervous laugh because seeing Jeff like that is so different than the way he was just a few weeks ago.

Sometimes, unexpectedly, Jeff's brain sends him signals to stand up from the wheelchair, but he can't, partly because he is still paralyzed on the left side and has an injured right knee, and partly because of the restraints. He grimaces and growls, fighting against the straps. It's hard to watch because I know him and see how frustrated he is to be tied to the chair, but I remind myself and everyone else in the family that it's all progress and better than seeing him lie in a bed with his eyes closed, doing nothing. Now he wants to do what would be normal for an eighteen-year-old, to take charge of his own body, and it saddens me that he can't, that he is no longer a normal eighteen-year-old.

It's now week four and I'm beginning to worry about keeping my job because I have not been to work in a month. So I make a rare appearance at my office. I'm happy to see everyone and to have a little bit of normalcy apart from the antiseptic smells and crisp white sheets world of the hospital. I get a lot of hugs and well wishes from people and it feels like just what I have needed but didn't even know I needed. I am happy to be at my desk rummaging through papers and checking messages when I get a phone call from the hospital social worker who I still have not met in person.

"We need to talk," she says. "It's time to start Jeff's discharge planning and discuss moving him to a comprehensive brain injury rehabilitation program."

I am taken by surprise and tears instantly come to my eyes. The idea of more hospitals is something I am not prepared for and I'm angry that she would spring this on me over the phone.

"No, I want to bring him home," I say. "And why would you tell me this over the phone when I haven't even met you?"

A part of me knows I am being unfair to her; she's just doing her job. But I'm getting used to pushing back with medical people who seem insensitive, and she's a social worker so I expect more from her. Steve and I meet with her the next day and I still don't like her but I am beginning to understand the need for a specialized brain injury program, and that Jeff is not ready to come home.

"You are so lucky," she tells us, "because you have good insurance that will cover it. A lot of people don't." She smiles and hands us the lucky people list of hospitals and addresses. "You get to choose from among the A list of rehabilitation hospitals!" she says as if she's just told us we won a trip to Bermuda.

The A list? I am more than a little shocked at the idea of different lists of options for different people based on their luck, their financial or social status. But if that's the way it is I am grateful to have the better options and for once I appreciate that Steve is in the military since that seems to be why we have the A list available to us. The Army has nothing to offer for intensive inpatient brain injury rehabilitation so they will pay for a private rehabilitation hospital.

As we prepare for moving Jeff to a rehabilitation hospital Steve has decided that's his cue to move out of our house. He has moved back to his apartment, once again living with Cynthia and her kids. At first he told me she was gone but I'm about a hundred years older and wiser than I was a month ago, so I demanded he take me over there to see that she no longer lived there. Sure enough her clothes were in his closet and her personal things in the bathroom. We came back to the house and had the worst fight ever that night, and then he left. So far as I'm concerned for the last time.

It's not fun for me that Steve and I have to coordinate to work out meeting at the places on the A list, but I will do it for Jeff. Steve and I set up tours of the hospitals in the Washington DC area and discuss the pros and cons of each, which only takes a couple of days because there are only two good options. The third best choice is in Pennsylvania and that seems to us to be too far away.

First we visit the brain injury and stroke unit of Mount Vernon Hospital in Alexandria, Virginia and next we tour a new brain injury unit at the National Rehabilitation Hospital in the northeast part of DC. We are not excited about either one so we meet with a group of doctors and a social worker at Walter Reed, but they are honest and tell us that what we thought is correct; the military has no such thing as a brain injury program like Jeff needs. They strongly suggest we take a look at the hospital in Pennsylvania.

"What should we look for?" I ask.

"I think a good certified rehabilitation nurse (CRN) is key because that CRN will be with him every day and can make a huge difference in his recovery," one doctor says. That makes sense to me and we set up an appointment to visit Bryn Mawr Rehabilitation Hospital in Malvern, Pennsylvania. They were selected that year as the number one rehabilitation hospital in the country.

We both know the minute we drive onto the grounds of Bryn Mawr that this is it. The hospital is surrounded by acres of beautiful pastoral land with horses grazing on the property. We learn as we tour the facility that they have a specialized brain injury unit for people who have recently come out of a coma, with a lot of people in Jeff's age group, and that their treatment teams work together in a coordinated and integrated manner. The woman giving us the tour describes their social and recreational activities and I know Jeff would enjoy that a lot. I just wish it wasn't so far away because I can't visit him every day, but we make our decision and Steve and I sign the paperwork to allow Bryn Mawr staff to do their assessment and begin the process of transferring Jeff there.

When we get home and visit Jeff we find the hospital has moved him out of the trauma ward to a standard medical unit upstairs, and when we visit him he is disoriented and upset with being in a different place. The nurses on that unit seem to be afraid of him and are understaffed to take care of him so now it's urgent that we move him to Bryn Mawr, but we have to wait for the transfer to be arranged and insurance to be worked out.

Meanwhile Jeff is more alert and growing more confused and agitated every day. The nurses say he's a problem and have documented in his medical records that he's "combative" and tried to bite one of them. They don't want to change his diapers so Steve has begun changing him so he doesn't develop bed sores, and we both do what we can to take care of him when we are there. I am still doing speech therapy with Jeff and he has begun speaking in short sentences. We have bizarre conversations and I love every second of them.

I know that a few of Jeff's teachers came in to see him over the weekend because they left balloons and cards, and one was from his third year Spanish teacher. She must have spoken to him in Spanish because after their visit Jeff was speaking Spanish and asking, "¿Por qué?" over and over.

When the nurses heard him speaking Spanish they thought he was fluent and wrote in his chart that he spoke Spanish and is bilingual. I think that's very strange because although he is good at languages, he is not bilingual and our family speaks only English.

Jeff has begun saying phrases that worry me like, "leave Jeff alone." I know he must be very frightened and I can't explain things to him, so I just want him to go somewhere that can give him the help he needs to begin healing and making sense of his new life. We need to get him transported. Pronto!

On March 20, 1989 Jeff is transported by ambulance to Bryn Mawr. Steve rides in the ambulance with Jeff, who is strapped onto a gurney in a semi-sitting position facing the back window so that he can watch me as I drive along behind them in my rental car. He grins and waves at me as if he thinks it's funny that I am in a car driving behind them. I am reminded of when he started preschool in Frankfurt and I stood in the snow holding Travis and smiling encouragement to four-year-old Jeff, who waved to me from the bus window.

Here we go, I think. Off to the next part of this adventure. Not what I planned to be doing this spring but hey, I'm beginning to get it; I have no control over my life at all.

The tricky part about rehabilitation after a brain injury is that you have to have patience and no patience all at the same time.

—Jeff Bouck, TBI Survivor

Chapter 3

Jeff Eats Green French Fries

WHEN WE ARRIVE AT BRYN MAWR, the Admissions director greets us and introduces us to a friendly rehabilitation nurse named Mary. Mary shows us to Jeff's room and helps him settle in, explaining things to him in simple language but with a respectful tone appropriate for the young adult he is. She tells him where he is and who she is, and he watches her intently. I can tell that Jeff likes Mary, and I instantly love her for the compassionate way she deals with him. Privately, Mary tells us more about Jeff's program and what to expect, and she shows us around the locked unit where other patients are in wheelchairs, beds, or walking with the help of therapists. The patients are mostly young, around Jeff's age, and the atmosphere is lively; it does not carry the depressing feel of the acute care hospital.

I understand now why the doctors at Walter Reed advised us that an experienced certified rehabilitation nurse is an important key to the success of a brain injury program. I feel so guilty leaving Jeff there, like I'm abandoning him, but the doctor in charge has explained to me that Jeff is at a stage in his recovery that requires professional involvement more than my presence. I want to trust them, and I think I can, but it's so hard after being with him every day since February 17.

"He's eighteen years old and this is his journey that he has to do himself," Mary tells me.

I know intellectually that I am not being a bad mother leaving him there, but it feels like it. I promise Jeff I will be back very soon and we leave him at Bryn Mawr, driving home with me in tears the whole way.

During his first week at Bryn Mawr, the rehabilitation team uses a variety of tools to assess Jeff's situation, including the Rancho Los Amigos (RLA) Scale of cognitive functioning. They explain that the RLA is a communication tool used among medical and rehabilitation professionals to describe how someone is functioning after a brain injury. He is determined to be at an RLA level of four.

This level is described in the information I am given as "Confused/ Agitated: Maximal Assistance." That means he needs a lot of assistance with everything, and as his brain heals he has become confused and therefore agitated. Agitation, the neuropsychologist tells me, is really the flip side of confusion and is a sign of progress. The characteristics and behaviors of someone at an RLA level of four are listed as:

- Alert and in heightened state of activity
- Purposeful attempts to remove restraints or tubes or crawl out of bed
- May perform motor activities such as sitting, reaching, and walking but without any apparent purpose or upon another's request
- Very brief and usually non-purposeful moments of sustained alternatives and divided attention
- Absent short-term memory
- May cry out or scream out of proportion to stimulus even after its removal
- May exhibit aggressive or flight behavior

- Mood may swing from euphoric to hostile with no apparent relationship to environmental events
- Unable to cooperate with treatment efforts
- Verbalizations are frequently incoherent and/or inappropriate to activity or environment

Steve and I are barely speaking now that he is once again living with his fake family at his apartment, so the plan we have developed is that I will be at Bryn Mawr on the weekends and one day a week so I can participate in Jeff's therapies and team meetings. The rest of the time I can go back to work and the rest of my life. Steve says he will come to visit Jeff when he can. I explain to Mary about our family problems and she is sympathetic and says she will make sure Jeff is well cared for.

Decisions about Jeff's care are falling entirely on me now and I am afraid I'll make the wrong decisions or that people will treat him badly when I'm not there and he won't be able to tell me. He is so vulnerable and it's so hard to know what is right. Even if I made the right choice moving him to a place so far from home, his friends can't visit and I can't be with him all of the time.

The first big, difficult decision I have to make is whether or not to let the doctors insert a gastrointestinal tube, or G tube, directly into Jeff's stomach because he is not eating and is losing weight. I don't think I realized how much weight he's lost but they tell me it's over forty pounds since his accident and he was on the thin side to begin with. The doctor tells me the NG tube, put in him when he was first hospitalized, was meant to be temporary and does not allow them to feed him enough liquid food. They say if I don't let them do this, Jeff will starve to death. They tested him for dysphagia, a swallowing disorder, and said he was medically cleared to eat but his brain isn't ready.

I don't see what the problem is; I don't get it. Why won't he eat when he's hungry? Mary waits patiently as I set out to prove them wrong, as I get Jeff in his wheelchair and put a tray of food in front of him. I explain to him that he has to eat, that he has lost a lot of weight, and I show him how to pick up a fork and spoon like I did when he was a baby learning to feed himself. I always encouraged my sons to do things independently and am determined he can do this. Jeff stares at me, grinning, nodding his head as if he understands, but he does not pick up his fork to eat. I keep trying until we both are frustrated and I am forced to accept what I don't want to know. His brain is just not ready and I finally understand and accept that the Bryn Mawr staff is right. I am learning quickly that I do not know as much about brain injury as I thought I did, and I agree to sign the papers.

After I am home on Sunday night I have nightmares about the G tube procedure planned for the next day. They told me he will be awake during the procedure but he won't know what's going on. I am horrified by the image of them doing that to him and him not understanding what's happening. Will he feel pain? Will he hate me for letting them do this to him? For some reason the decision to let them insert a G tube is another wake-up call that this is going to be a long and difficult journey. I hang onto the knowledge that Mary will take care of him and that helps me to feel better.

Jeff has started to call Mary "Primary Nurse" which Steve and I were both confused about until we saw that is what it says on her name tag. We laughed and then we cried because we realized he is beginning to be able to read again. Jeff can read!

Jeff being away at a brain injury rehabilitation hospital is not at all like him going to college but I pretend it is so that I don't feel the guilt of abandoning him to strangers. And I am grateful for the opportunity to have some of my own life back and to have time again with Travis. I know I've neglected him and I'm worried because his grades have plummeted. We have had no structure to our home life, and he's been on his own so much that sometimes he's resistant when I try to parent him now, but I know this has been so hard on him so I give him a lot of slack. Or maybe it's because I'm too tired to fight with him.

The other good thing about Jeff being at Bryn Mawr is that during the week I'm able to go back to a semi-normal routine and be on campus at least a few days each week. What I've worked out is that I go to Gallaudet Monday, Wednesday, Thursday, and Friday mornings. On Tuesdays and on Saturdays and Sundays I drive back-and-forth to Pennsylvania to be with Jeff.

Travis goes with me only every other weekend so that he can have some social life of his own, and on the alternate weekends Steve has said he will stay at the house with him or have him over to his apartment. But that just isn't happening and even though Travis says he's fine by himself on those weekends when I'm gone, I worry. After all, he says, he's used to it and besides he has his friends and a part-time job to keep him busy. This is all true but not the same as having a parent at home, which I know all teenagers need even when they think they don't. I have no choice but to give in and just hope he doesn't get into trouble.

When I first showed up at Suburban Hospital without Steve, just before moving to Bryn Mawr, I told Jeff that his dad and I would not be coming to visit together anymore because Steve was back with Cynthia. Jeff looked at me wide-eyed and grinned.

"He's got holes in his head where he should have brains," he said in the sing-song voice that had become his new way of speaking.

Travis and I had a good laugh over that. The way Jeff is speaking now is funny, sometimes with great insight but with those weird inflections and sentence constructions that sound like he's in a cartoon.

Last Tuesday I got to Bryn Mawr and Jeff was still in bed. He looked happy to see me and gave me a big wave and lopsided grin.

Then in his new lyrical way of talking he sang out, "Jeff would like to say to the person he commonly calls Mother, hello!"

Translation: Hi Mom!

Next he came out with the convoluted sentence: "Jeff would love for the person he constantly calls, oh, Mother, to tell the persons he calls friends that Jeff would love for the persons he calls friends to visit."

Translation: Tell my friends to visit me!

As a speech-language pathologist I was curious why Jeff talked in third person about himself as he's redeveloping his expressive language and self-awareness so I asked the neuropsychologist, who I really like, why? She suggested it might be a form of psychological detachment; identifying too closely with this damaged person is so painful. But I also think maybe it's the reemergence of his metacognition, thinking about thinking, because Jeff always did study people in a slightly detached, intellectual sort of way. I know him better than they do and sometimes I see things differently than the therapists do. This is a good place though because they listen to me and welcome me as part of the rehabilitation team. We are all working together to help Jeff.

Jeff is working in physical therapy and occupational therapy to relearn how to use his hands, propel his wheelchair around the unit, sit up, and do very basic activities. Some days I help and have patience but other days I'm anxious for him to get back to normal and I get frustrated. I admire the staff at Bryn Mawr because they never show frustration; they are always patient with these people. Yesterday I was especially exasperated by his reluctance to eat because I know that means he will continue to need the G tube. I can't imagine dealing with that when I bring him home.

Travis and their friend Jon were with me and Jon decided to try to help get Jeff to eat. Jeff was sitting on the edge of his bed with a tray in front of him, staring at green beans on his plate and refusing to eat them.

"Hey man, they're just green French fries!" Jon told him. Jeff laughed and ate the green beans.

So I learned something important that day. You just never know what will work with someone who has a TBI! If I ever go back to doing clinical work I think I'll have a lot more insight and ideas about how to help people after going through this journey with Jeff.

May 1989

IT'S BEEN A COUPLE OF MONTHS since our rehabilitation adventure began and Jeff is making a lot of progress. But he has started asking more questions about why he's at Bryn Mawr, and when he will go home. I don't know what to tell him so I just say "soon" and encourage him to work hard in his therapy. He looks at me like he doesn't trust me. I have been told it's a part of his brain healing. His perceptions are mistaken but he believes them and thinks the rest of us have brain damage.

Most of the patients on his unit believe they have been captured and we—family members and staff—are all in a conspiracy to keep them as hostages. It's funny to hear them making plans to escape and it's perfectly normal to open the door to the locked unit, using the password, and find someone in a wheelchair, strategically placed behind the door waiting to sneak out when anyone opens it. Like we wouldn't notice them! They're all like Jeff, adults seated in wheelchairs but acting and looking like children in their sweatpants, adult diapers, and T-shirts.

The hardest part is when Jeff is depressed or angry. One weekend the nurses said he was talking about blowing up the place or jumping out of his second story window. Another day, after he began walking with a lot of assistance, I got permission to take him out for a drive and wheeled him out to the parking lot. As we got close to the car, he began to cry out and yell, saying he hated himself and what he had become, and that he knew he would never walk again. I reminded him that he had started to walk in therapy but he needed the wheelchair for safety because we were going out for the afternoon.

"I know you're all lying to me saying that I'll get better," he yelled. "I don't want to live like this, in a wheelchair!" My heart was breaking as I listened to him.

"Jeff, you are making progress," I told him racking my brain for something to say. "And if you think about it, it's a good thing that you are becoming depressed!"

That got his attention. He stared at me with rage in his eyes. I kept talking even though I wasn't sure I was saying the right things. "It's a good sign because that means your brain is healing and you are aware of more!"

That really made him mad.

"You think it's good I can't walk!" he screamed at the top of his voice. "You think it's progress that I want to die!" He looked at me like I was his enemy.

"Jeff, of course not!" I said trying to hug him, but he pulled away from me.

We had an all-out yelling match right there in the parking lot but finally he just stopped abruptly and said he could see what I meant. What changed his mind? I'll never know. Maybe he just forgot what he was arguing about, or maybe some ability to use logic suddenly woke up. Whatever it was, we went out for a drive and stopped at McDonalds and had a nice afternoon together. And after that I saw him working even harder.

I love my days with Jeff. When I'm at Bryn Mawr I meet with therapists and participate in his physical, occupational, speech-language, and recreation therapy sessions and for the most part being there helps me to stay aware that he is making small incremental steps toward nearly normal functioning. He's walking and talking, and some days he seems alert and almost like his old self. I feel at home when I'm there, maybe even more than when I am at my house in Maryland, especially when I'm talking to other family members and the nurses.

At the end of May the Bryn Mawr staff holds a discharge planning meeting to go over all of the therapy Jeff will need when he comes home. This meeting is a big deal, so Travis goes with me, and we all sit in a room waiting for Steve to show up too. He never does, so we go on without him. I leave feeling like we have a plan in place, but I feel a little guilty that I wasn't one hundred percent honest with them. I didn't mention that I will need surgery sometime over the summer; I don't want them to get involved with that or think I can't handle things. I just want Jeff to come home.

Even though we have a plan now, and I'm happy Jeff will be back with us, I'm scared. For one thing he still has his G tube and the doctors told me also that he might need to have a walker or wheelchair in case he is still having trouble walking, because he's not steady all of the time. I'm seeing that this is going to be a long, slow recovery process for some time after Jeff leaves Bryn Mawr. Jeff is excited about leaving and to him it's way past time.

One day I visit him and find that he has pulled his G tube out. He has decided he doesn't need it any more. He has folded it up neatly and put it on a shelf and I have to laugh because this is so like Jeff to take charge of things and go against medical advice. He's still very thin but he is eating better so the staff agrees that we can leave it out and I'm relieved.

June 1989

FINALLY, THE LONG-AWAITED DAY comes to bring my son home. It's been over four months since he was first injured and transported to Suburban Hospital. Four long months that have changed everything in my life.

All month the staff at Bryn Mawr has worked to get Jeff ready for this day, for the transition back to home. On June 28, 1989, I get up early and drive north through the rain on Interstate 95, not thinking of anything much except that I am going to Pennsylvania to bring Jeff back to our house in Maryland. I am so excited to start getting our family back to normal. I'm still furious with Steve for not showing up for the discharge planning meeting, so I don't even tell him Jeff is coming home. If he calls me, which I don't expect, I'll tell him Jeff's back so he can visit him. It's his own fault he's out of the loop.

I arrive at Bryn Mawr to find Jeff sitting on his bed in the small apartment he was moved to as part of a transitional program to prepare him for returning home. He's mad about something, and as we talk I learn that it's his roommate, a guy the same age as Jeff.

"What are you mad at him for?" I ask.

"He just acts so brain-injured!" he says. He complains some more about the things his roommate has done and said, all similar to what Jeff does and says all the time, and then announces he's ready to leave. I ask the psychologist about Jeff's problem with his roommate and she says it's normal; it's like looking in a mirror and he doesn't like what he sees. Plus they are the same age and highly competitive.

I sign paperwork for his release and help him to finish packing. I'm relieved that we are leaving the hospital without a wheelchair or a G tube and feeding equipment. We make the rounds, saying goodbye to other family members and all the staff who have helped us for three months. I am misty-eyed. It feels like saying goodbye to family and I know I'll miss these people and this place even if Jeff doesn't.

The staff has a small send-off party, complete with balloons and cards. We all applaud Jeff as he walks unassisted out the front entrance to our car parked in the semi-circular driveway. He beams with pride and happiness in a way I haven't seen for a long time. As he gets in the car he thanks people and waves.

Then his face turns serious. "Let's get out of here!" he says when I get into the driver's seat. "I hate this place!"

I guess I expected him to feel the same love and appreciation I do for the work the staff had done. But he has already told me many times in the past month that he hates it there, and I know what he really hates is what the hospital represents to him. He hates that he has damage to his brain, and he hates all of the problems that he has. Jeff with a brain injury is like an athlete who has lost the use of his arms or legs. The ability to be smart and independent was everything to Jeff and I know that he feels he has lost that.

I try to keep the conversation positive and upbeat but he sees the paperwork sitting in the front seat and insists on reading his discharge summary and the other reports. He laughs at some of it but becomes infuriated when he reads therapy notes that say he has "silly speech." I drive us out of the Bryn Mawr property, through the town of Malvern, and around the back roads to Interstate 95 heading home and listen to him go on and on about his complaints about Bryn Mawr and this report.

"What? They just don't understand my humor," he says.

"But Jeff, sometimes you do make silly jokes," I say.

Finally he moves on to other topics and I think about what his reaction means, how much he's going to be confronted with at home. He's going back to the world he used to live in as a different person, not as the same Jeff everyone knew before the brain injury. People will notice that he is silly at times and often very confused.

But I have my son back and that's all that matters to me. I'm singing as we travel down the highway listening to Jeff's favorite songs on the radio, and I fill him in on what's happening with his brother and the dog.

"Christy will be so happy to see you!" I say and he smiles. He has said many times that he missed the dog and wanted to see her. "And Travis is excited about having you home, and your friends will be coming to see you over the next few days."

We stop at the Maryland Rest Stop and Jeff is excited about the simple activity of visiting a place outside of the community surrounding Bryn Mawr. He's like an inmate who has just been released from prison. I buy him all the junk food he wants, and of course get the same for me. I'm still overeating but once Jeff is home I promised myself I will go on a diet.

As we near our home in Olney, Jeff asks if we can stop a few streets away and surprise a girl he has been friends with. I wait in the car and watch as he goes to her door, she answers, and they talk for a few minutes. He comes back to the car laughing. He says she was definitely surprised and she told him she had thought he was dead. That doesn't seem funny to me but to Jeff it is. I guess in an odd teenager way it makes him feel important to be the subject of dramatic rumors like that.

Travis is home when we arrive, and we celebrate Jeff's homecoming as a family. We order pizza and I'm happy to spend a peaceful evening with just Jeff, Travis, our dog Christy, and me. But I'm also apprehensive and unsure of how much to help Jeff get ready for bed. I'm worried about him going up and down the stairs. I'm afraid he'll fall, and I'm caught between wanting to take care of him like a child and knowing that he has to do things for himself. In therapy he relearned how to brush his teeth, put on pajamas, and all of those things we do on our own at night so I just remind him what to do and wait to say goodnight.

As we each go to our own rooms, I realize I am feeling hypervigilant. I lie awake for at least an hour listening for footsteps or for Jeff to call out from down the hall. I'm exhausted, but I can't go to sleep. Last year, before Jeff's TBI, I was diagnosed with PTSD from childhood trauma, and I have never been able to relax if I don't know where people are in the house.

I don't want to admit that I am afraid of my own son, but I am. He's a stranger; a tall and very thin brain-damaged young man who I know is confused and unpredictable. Will he wander from his room, be disoriented and fall down the stairs? Will he wake up confused about where he is and walk into my room? Will he try to leave the house in the middle of the night as he and Travis did too many times before?

Nothing unusual happens though, and the next morning I am in the kitchen when Jeff comes down, happy just to be making pancakes for my two sons again. It's Saturday and, as planned, Jeff's friends stop by to welcome him home. It's a thrill to see him with them again laughing and joking. But I notice the disconnect when he does not remember the things they want to talk about, things they've all done together or inside jokes.

The next day a few of Jeff's buddies, Travis, and Jon take him out to play putt-putt golf at a nearby course in Rockville. I watch the clock, only relaxing when they finally bring him home at the time they said they would. They are taking this role of helping Jeff seriously and I'm relieved to see that.

After Jeff's been home just a few days the doorbell rings and I open it to find two policemen on my porch there to arrest my son. His history of speeding and ignoring the associated traffic tickets has caught up with him in the legal system. This is not a total surprise because while he was at Suburban Hospital, and in a coma, Steve said the police had appeared one day while I was out of the room and tried to arrest Jeff then.

Steve thought it was funny, and told me he had laughed at them and said, "Sure go ahead, but you have to take all of his medical equipment with him!"

So they went away that day and I forgot all about it. Somewhere in the back of my mind I knew Jeff was driving with a suspended license when the accident happened, so I probably should have expected this. Now here is the long arm of the law reaching out to claim him and make him pay his debt to society. How ridiculous.

I stare at the two young men at the door.

"He has a severe traumatic brain injury and just got home from a rehabilitation hospital," I tell them. "He can't answer your questions." I just want them to disappear but they don't.

Despite my very clear explanations about his limitations, they insist that Jeff go with them in the police car, and I am told to follow along behind to the station.

Once there an officer explains to me that he has to take Jeff to a small room to question him. I insist on going along.

"He's eighteen years old mam, legally an adult, and that means you cannot go in there with him," he says.

I argue but he won't budge; it's the rule. So I laugh to myself and sit down in the waiting area, smug in knowing this will be quite the experience for that rather naive young policeman.

In under five minutes, they are back. The red-faced officer admits that I was right. Jeff could not remember anything and was unable to answer any questions. He wandered off-topic so much he was impossible to interview. Duh! We are free to go home but will be notified about a court hearing.

As our new normal life begins, I see daily evidence of how Jeff's cognitive impairments affect everything. I had heard of this but never could have imagined how hard it would be. Some of his old knowledge is there and some isn't, so I never know what's going to happen. Each day is different and every activity Jeff tries has unpredictable ups and downs. I'm constantly taken by surprise and kept off balance.

He remembers things from his favorite books, or phrases in Latin or Spanish, but he doesn't remember how to do simple activities such as make toast, use the microwave, or go out to the mailbox at the end of the driveway. I see that, even though he practiced activities of daily living (ADLs) in his rehabilitation therapies, our home is a different environment and his brain no longer generalizes what he learned at Bryn Mawr to these novel situations.

This is hard, almost too hard. I have to tell him obvious things over and over and it's mentally exhausting just keeping on top of what he's trying to do. I have to break everything down into small steps and when he does it wrong I have to show him what to do over and over and over and over. Travis has no patience for this, although he's trying, and I see him getting frustrated and disappointed.

Being Jeff's mom has reverted to the job it was when he was much younger, and I am stressed but I cannot let myself be angry at him. I just want so much to fix it all. When people I care about are hurting, it's normal for me to automatically become a helper, and this is my son so I obsess over ways to help him.

I have not found outpatient therapy programs yet so I am working overtime trying to think of things we can do at home that would help Jeff improve his cognitive abilities. I give him small tasks to do at first like help clear dishes from the table, or feed the dog, or help me do the grocery shopping. There are days I have to go to my room and cry because I am worried he will never be able to do these normal things for himself.

Jeff was always a cute kid and has become a handsome young man, but these days he often looks weird and smells bad. I finally realized that it's because he forgets to shave, shower, and use deodorant; I have to remind him and it embarrasses both of us. I don't know if people at Bryn Mawr even mentioned this but apparently Jeff lost his sense of smell with his TBI so he doesn't notice any body odor. Travis and I certainly do, though!

I try to keep my sense of humor about this but I don't want Jeff to be a social outcast when he's able to do more and be around people. He frequently shaves only part of his face and doesn't comb his hair, and some days he wears his shirt inside out or backward or both. On those off days he looks like that scary guy I might see on the street and immediately avoid.

"Jeff, you look like a homeless person," I say at those times.

He laughs and thinks it's a joke.

So I have to be more specific.

"Go comb your hair, and shave the other side of your face," I say.

He looks at me like I'm crazy. "I think I look fine."

"Go look in the mirror," I tell him, leading him to the hall bathroom. He glances in the bathroom mirror and still insists he looks fine. I am lost. How can I convince him of something he doesn't see, and how is it that his perceptions are so off that he can't see it? Or is it just rebellion?

63

When Travis is around I ask him to intervene because, after all, what eighteen-year-old guy wants his mom to help him get dressed? I know Travis will be direct with him because as a sixteen-year-old he does not want his brother going out looking like that.

"Dude, you look like hell," Travis says. Jeff laughs but when it's his brother telling him those things he pays attention. He lets Travis help him shave and dress better. I guess it's like the green bean "French fries" at Bryn Mawr.

It reminds me of when the kids were little and a four-year-old Jeff helped two-year-old Travis learn how to dress himself. Except now the roles are reversed. Travis is busy though and he can't always be there to help with Jeff.

I see that Jeff needs the ongoing outpatient therapy recommended in his discharge reports, but I don't know what to do. When we left Bryn Mawr the question of where to go for outpatient rehabilitation had not been completely resolved. I begin visiting the places on the list of recommended therapy facilities and programs. There is a physical therapy clinic near us in Olney, but they do not offer any of the other therapy he needs and do not specialize in brain injury. They are more into sports injuries.

I have no idea how I am going to put this all together for him in a way that will work for our family. Driving in the Washington DC area takes a lot of time and I simply cannot spend all day driving Jeff around to different locations in Montgomery County.

I have to work and Jeff needs constant supervision so I come up with a plan that I think will be perfect until I can figure out something better.

I make arrangements with Dave Martin to take Jeff to work with me at Gallaudet, thinking that he can get exercise walking around campus with me, and I can find things for him to do that would be like cognitive therapy. Dave is very understanding, partly because of his interest in the study of cognition. He has published a lot of articles and teaches classes on the topic.

Everyone in the office gets into this. We set Jeff up with a desk in the hall outside of my office and Dave even takes the time to work with him using a program called Instrumental Enrichment (IE). It's pretty interesting to me and I wonder if this might make a good dissertation topic. IE was developed for people with brain damage or mental retardation. It uses a visual system to organize dots into patterns that approximate the cognitive processes we all use for everything. Things like making comparisons, seeing patterns, understanding the concept of same and different, and so on. However, we quickly see that Jeff is not ready for this kind of activity because he is way too distractible and it only frustrates him.

The other problem with this arrangement is that I get very little work done because Jeff talks all the time! He has no filter anymore and his constant patter is too distracting to everyone around him, so I see this will not work even for just a month or so. This TBI thing, life after a brain injury, is completely different from anything I've ever experienced before. I am admitting defeat.

I begin making calls to places on the list that Bryn Mawr staff gave me. I am determined to find the perfect brain injury day treatment program for Jeff, and am convinced he deserves nothing but the best. I can't find anything though, and I find myself in tears one day as I hang up the phone from inquiring about yet another program that just doesn't fit.

I am on the edge of panic and hysteria as I call a social worker at the National Rehabilitation Hospital, and she gives me the best advice of anyone.

"You know, you just can't do it perfectly," she says after listening to our story. "It's not possible."

I burst into tears. I see now that I have to look for something that's "good enough" instead of the absolute best program. Perfect is probably not out there. And I'm running out of time to find it because soon I will be in the hospital myself.

I call the case manager assigned to us for CHAMPUS, the Army's outpatient insurance plan, and with her help I finally find a specialized brain injury day program that focuses on cognitive therapy and gives Jeff a place to go during the day. It's not perfect—they don't have physical or occupational therapy—but they do have an arrangement with another program and they provide transportation services back-and-forth. They will also work with the school system to help Jeff finish the one class he needs for high school. I met with the school counselor and was surprised to learn Jeff had finished all of his required classes during his junior year and all he was taking was advanced classes and electives except for English.

I guess I am lucky—there's that word again—to have this resource available because the director of the program had been involved for years with the state Head Injury Association in Maryland and she knows how to help work out the payments through a combination of CHAMPUS and some state funding, and somehow it will even cover taxi service to and from our house every day so I don't have to drive him there.

That's one thing off my plate, and I am relieved, because I am exhausted. I know that it isn't just depression making me tired all of the time and that it's also because my illness, whatever it is, is getting worse.

While Jeff was at Bryn Mawr, just before I brought him home, my doctor ignored my protests and scheduled a partial hysterectomy for mid-August.

"You have a tumor in your uterus and we can't see your ovaries, so we don't know until we open you up how much we will have to take out," she said.

I cried and gave her my whole sob story about why I couldn't do that, but in the end she just said I had no choice. I've been avoiding thinking about it and I'm panicked about what to do with the kids. At least now I have Jeff in a good day program, but I have to get

Steve's help and I hate that because I don't trust him. Besides, we are just not talking anymore except through lawyers.

I have to make the call though, so I try him at work. He says of course he will take care of Jeff and Travis, as if there is no question, as if I've imagined all of the months that he has been absent from our lives. I'm worried about Cynthia and her kids being around because Jeff gets rattled so easily and there's too much chaos and too many people in that small apartment. So I tell Steve she and her kids have to move out while Jeff and Travis are there, which is only going to be about a week. He says he will tell her that.

About my TBI, imagine that there is a person with a GIANT paintbrush who follows me through life. EVERY time I have an experience this person waits until it is over and quickly paints over it.

—Jeff Bouck, TBI Survivor

Chapter 4

My Life Needs a New Script

August 1989

AS I PREPARE TO GO into the hospital for my hysterectomy I realize I can no longer take care of our dog, Christy, because I am too sick and have too many responsibilities, and no energy. I ask Steve to take care of her and he, of course, says no. I'm left with only one option, so with a sinking heart, I try to find Christy a new home. She has become a behavior problem. She regularly uses the living room carpet as the great outdoors so our whole house smells of dog pee, and I cannot get rid of the odor no matter how hard I try. When I go to pick her up now she often snarls at me, probably because I've been yelling at her so often for peeing in the house. It's not fair to her to keep her with us when there is no one to care for her or play with her.

On a sad day, about a week before I check in to the hospital, I give the dog a bath and brush her fluffy coat of hair to make her as cute as possible, and then Jeff, Travis and I take Christy to the county humane society to be placed for adoption. I cry all the way there, but I know she is not happy with us and none of us are too thrilled with her behavior anymore either.

I do my best for Christy, lying on the intake forms, giving her good marks for being completely housebroken, and I check the box that says she has no behavioral issues. It is all in how you look at it, isn't it? Her behavior is not her fault, just a reflection of our family dysfunction; she deserves a stable home. I feel sure if she gets that she will go back to being the wonderful family pet she has been for us for four years.

As I stand at the front counter, filling out the paperwork, a family with two small children comes in and I see Christy scrunch down, wag her tail, and wiggle her way across the floor to the kids as if on cue. It's as if she knows she needs a new family too.

"Oh Mommy, look how cute she is!" the little boy says. Whew. I call the next day and am told she had been adopted right away. They can't tell me who it was but I hope it was that family who came in while I was filling out the paperwork. I picture her being loved and played with by those children, happy in her new home, and then I put her out of my mind.

I have a long list of things to do before surgery. I was told I would be unable to drive or go to work for about six weeks, so I meet with my Department Chair, Dr. Bill Marshall, and with Dave to explain that I will have to be out again. They are willing to do what they can to help me, and grant me a year's extension on finishing my dissertation. However, I lose my job. Dave is apologetic but I have barely been at work for the past six months and now it will be even longer, so I understand. It is unreasonable to expect that the university will continue to pay me when I can't do the work. Dave offers me a small contract to continue doing a newsletter along with some other writing and editing from home and I am grateful to have at least that much. The truth is that I am kind of relieved to get fired because I am so tired that, even though I am afraid to face the prospect of having no job, I just want to lie down somewhere and rest for about a year. I have to accept that I cannot do it all anymore.

The doctors call surgery "going under the knife," which brings up visions of the movie Psycho, and the images give me nightmares. I console myself by focusing on the future, thinking that this surgery will be over soon and I will soon be home to take care of my kids and go on with my life. I can't even think about the financial challenges I know are waiting just around the corner. I will figure out later what to do about being unemployed; for now I just have to get through this.

My doctor wakes me up right after the surgery to tell me I have ovarian cancer and that they had to do a complete hysterectomy after all. She says something about how she wanted me to hear it from her which makes no sense to me at that awful moment. I hear the words ovarian cancer and think I am going to die.

I begin screaming "No!" and they put me back to sleep.

I wake up sometime later in the worst physical pain I've ever felt, even worse than labor or what I remember of being run over by a car when I was a child. I am also more afraid than I have ever been. I have ovarian cancer; people always die from that don't they? Who will take care of Jeff and Travis if I die?

Be a good girl, and be quiet, my father used to tell me. He and my mother told the story about how I would repeat his words when I was two years old.

They said I would say: "Janny good girl; didn't scream; didn't holler; didn't fuss."

So I don't tell anyone my fears. I feel like I am living in a bad movie where the main character keeps having one over-the-top obstacle after another thrown at her. Except that this isn't a movie at all. It's my real life. My doctor says that they do not know yet what type of ovarian cancer I have. Type? I didn't know ovarian cancer came in different flavors. She says it will take some time to get the lab results back and her words of advice for me are to "hope for the best but prepare for the worst."

That sounds familiar.

It's the same thing they told me when Jeff had his car accident.

It takes eight very long days for the lab at Walter Reed to complete their analysis and during that time I lie in that hospital bed glad to be high on morphine. I bargain with a God I am not even sure I believe in anymore. It is obvious that I am going to have to ask for help, even though I am no good at it and have no idea who to ask. I am estranged from my family of origin and feel I have no parents in my life anymore and now no husband. I feel I have no family at all except for my children and they are young and also broken; they are on overload themselves even if they don't know it. I have never felt so completely abandoned and frightened in my life.

My running monologue with a deity vaguely familiar from my traditional Christian upbringing in my childhood goes something like this: "God, if you are there, please help me and I will change my life. I promise. I know I have made a lot of mistakes and I will do everything I can to take better care of myself and my sons if you let me live. I will change my life. I promise. I'll do whatever you want me to do." I wait for a response.

That small voice inside of me, the one that had recently begun to speak up, reminds me that the only way to make those changes is to make the hard choices that for years had scared me into inaction. But things are very different now and I am at last willing to do whatever it takes.

It seems that the intense, relentless trauma that has kept coming at me has accomplished something that nothing else ever could have; it has knocked me into a new state of knowing what is important and what isn't. Priorities are clearer than they have ever been; they are now written in bright neon, glowing paint on my hospital walls. As Dr. Stone has told me, I have to put myself first.

It's all about changing my relationships, including my relationship to myself. Some people I have tried to be close to in the past, like Steve, I now have to let go of. And I have to learn how to take better care of myself and not betray myself all of the time by saying I don't need what I know inside I do need. I have always thought of myself as an honest person but maybe I'm not because I have not been honest with myself. Dr. Stone says I go for the opposite of what I want. How crazy is that? He also says that was why I didn't trust myself; I am not trustworthy to me. That's the bottom line. It's why I always felt so guilty, and not for the reasons my mother told me. She always said my migraine headaches and other problems were from what she called a "deep seated guilt" because I had always been hostile toward her. That led me to a lifetime of trying to prove to her that I loved her, which was a trap.

I see that my self-neglect is what has always made me feel that unexplainable guilt. I can see it clearly now, but I don't know how I will ever change it because I have lived my whole life focusing on the needs of other people. Still, I have to try. And I have to start now.

It strikes me that this is truly a life and death situation; my life and Jeff's are hanging by a thread and I have to take full responsibility for my own health and happiness, pushing away anything that distracts me from that mission. I am learning that no matter how much I wish it were different, there is simply no one else to do that for me. Of course knowing these things is different than being able to do them, and I don't know if I have the strength. I have to try though.

Breathing deeply, I pick up the hospital phone and do something uncomfortable and new.

I call my friend Judy, who is visiting her parents in New Jersey for the end of the summer. I tell her I need someone there, and confess that I am scared and feel completely alone with all of this.

"I'll do whatever you need," she says. I cry tears of relief and shock when I realize that it is really that simple to ask for support and have someone give it to me.

Judy comes home a few days early and spends her days with me at the hospital. Gradually other people find out where I am and they show up to sit by my bedside and cheer me up, too. I begin to realize I have a lot of friends after all. They sympathize with me, and entertain me by singing songs or blowing up the hospital's rubber gloves into balloons to bat around the room.

The doctors decide I should have blood transfusions to build me up for chemo therapy in case I need it. As the nurse gets me ready for the blood transfusions, I am literally shaking and my blood pressure goes through the roof. I want my kids with me but Steve is late bringing them to the hospital.

I call his apartment to see where he is and Cynthia answers the phone.

"Why are you there?" I yell at her. "Steve promised me you would leave so that he could take care of our kids!"

With an air of entitlement, she says. "Because I live here."

I slam the phone down.

I am panicked and enraged. How could Steve do this? He knows that Jeff cannot handle that level of confusion, and I also know now from Travis that Cynthia drinks a lot, smokes pot, and does cocaine. I do not want either of my kids around someone who uses drugs. Plus the part of this scenario that enrages me the most is that this is just not what we, Steve and I, had agreed to. But then that is why we are not together, isn't it? He always does whatever he wants to rather than what we agree to.

I lie in the hospital bed waiting for Steve to show up so I can yell at him. I am not going to be a good girl anymore and keep silent. All I can think of is that once again Steve is putting this other woman and her kids ahead of our family's needs, and as the nurse hooks me up to machines for the transfusion I cry and tell her what's going on.

"You're not going to confront him here are you?" she asks me with big eyes, looking like a scared puppy.

"Damn right I am!" I say.

"Your blood pressure is dangerously high," she says. "You need to relax."

When you are angry, really angry, and someone tells you to relax it does not help you to relax at all. "Then let me yell at my husband!"

I scream. She nods and moves the other woman who is in there out to a different room. I guess I scare them?

When Steve calmly walks into the room, with his usual demeanor of "everything's fine," I have tubes of blood circulating from a transfusion machine next to my bed, into my arm, and back again. His sister is with him and she takes one look at me, sees all of that blood, and turns green. As she leaves the room looking sick I wonder what Steve had told her was going on. Maybe she expected me to be sitting in the bed with a nice cup of tea, ready for a visit?

"You bastard! Our son has a brain injury and I have cancer!" I yell. "You goddamn son of a bitch!" I do not have an eloquent speech prepared.

Steve looks at me with his wide-eyed innocent gaze, and asks me, "Why are you so upset?"

I lose the tiny bit of composure I have been holding onto and resume yelling at the top of my lungs, knowing that the only way out of my rage is straight through it.

"You promised! You can't have Jeff there with all that confusion! You promised you wouldn't do this!"

"Jeff is fine," he says and then he tells me, as if it sounds perfectly reasonable, that he had arranged for Jeff and Travis to stay by themselves in an apartment near his. It's in the same complex and belongs to a friend who had gone on vacation. See? No problem!

I laugh now, struck by how funny he is, or at least how funny it would have been if the situation were not so serious.

All my life I have been told by my father that I am crazy and overly emotional, but now that little voice inside of me is getting stronger and saying, "Look! He's the crazy one, not you." And it feels great to know that.

I ignore him and turn to the nurse cowering in the corner. I tell her I have to see my kids and she goes to get them. Travis comes in first and says he's okay, but when he leaves and the nurse escorts Jeff to my bedside, he becomes very rattled seeing me with tubes of blood coming out of me, and he starts saying things that do not make any sense. The nurse watches us closely and after Steve leaves she quietly tells me that, after seeing and hearing Jeff, she now understands. She agrees to contact the hospital social worker right away. I want to kiss her.

The hospital social worker shows up later that morning and sits by my bed to listen as I explain about Jeff's brain injury and how worried I am about him being with Steve. Thanks to the military's top-down structure, which I never liked before, Steve is forced to move Cynthia and her children out of his apartment until I am able to go home. Finally, I am able to relax and focus on sleeping and healing while I wait to find out my fate.

When the lab reports come back, I get the good news that I have an "ovarian cancer of low malignancy potential." I had never heard of that, but in essence it means the cancer is not aggressive. My doctor says that the cancer had spread to my abdomen but removing the primary site, my ovaries, would stop it from spreading further. I will need to be followed for the next year but should eventually be okay and will not need chemo therapy after all. And the really good news is that I am not going to die.

About a week later, on the day I am discharged from Walter Reed, Steve picks me up from the hospital and drives me to the house. He carries my things to what used to be our bedroom and tells me he can't stay because he is meeting Cynthia for lunch.

"When I just got home from the hospital?" I ask. I want to talk to him about a lot of things, including a plan for us getting a divorce, and here he's running off again.

"She's having health problems," he says with a sincere look of worry. "She has a cyst on her ovaries and they are worried it might burst."

Oh dear. Poor Cynthia has a cyst. Her cyst trumps my ovarian cancer?

There is no question in my mind anymore that our marriage is definitely over. I have to keep my bargain with God and move on, and for the first time I want to.

"It was supposed to be for better or worse," I tell him.

"Well, I just couldn't do it," he says. That may be the first truthful thing he has told me in a long time.

I ask him why, in all the years we had been together, he had never asked me how I felt about anything. He thinks for a minute, pondering my question as if it is an interesting intellectual exercise.

"I guess I didn't really want to know," he says. "I assumed I wouldn't like the answer."

Well, that explains a lot! I feel stupid for believing all those years, since we were seventeen years old, that he did care. I tell him to leave and then I climb in bed and cry myself to sleep until the boys get home at the end of the day.

I have a comfortable master bedroom to camp out in with a king-sized bed and a television, an adjoining bathroom, and bottles of soda and snacks stashed nearby. The only problem is the stairs. I can't go up and down stairs and the kitchen is on the first floor, while our bedrooms are on the second. The kids do what they can to help me but Travis is starting his junior year of high school and Jeff is off to his outpatient rehabilitation program every day. So I am forced to ask for help once again. I reached out to my friends, and once again to my surprise they show up to help.

People come to the house and cook or bring me take-out food, and the days pass until I can take care of myself. As I heal physically I have a lot of time to think, and I cannot wait to be divorced and move on to healing in more ways than just from Jeff's TBI and my ovarian cancer.

I feel free of so much that has been holding me back in life; I am no longer stuck in a sick marriage, or the old fantasy that a man would take care of me. I look forward to being single. It's so much better to be single and lonely than to be married and lonely, I decide, and I no longer trust that the Hallmark Family I grew up wanting even exists. Instead of being Cinderella looking for Prince Charming I want to be the heroine in a new movie about me, a woman who takes charge of her life.

EVER SINCE I WAS A CHILD, autumn has been my favorite time of the year, and in the bustling metropolis of Washington DC it is an exciting time, the air full of possibilities. The fall season brings fresh starts and new beginnings, and I get an energetic and exciting sensation that something big is about to happen. Maybe it's because I loved the start of school, meeting new friends, and getting out of the house after a long, usually boring summer. Autumn weather is crisp and cooling from the muggy August heat; the leaves are turning red and golden and decorate the streets. Best of all, the tourists have gone home so it is possible to visit the Smithsonian museums or stroll through the streets of DC or the suburbs in the evening to one of the many wonderful restaurants or theaters.

But in the fall of 1989, I am not able to enjoy anything like I used to. I have no idea what the future holds for me and my kids. It feels like I am traveling to an unclear destination with a road map that has been rained on and partially destroyed. To top it off, there is a tornado on the horizon. I live in fear of the next bad thing happening. It seems like my life keeps changing for the worse no matter what I do. I tell Dr. Stone I feel like I am climbing a mountain and every time I get somewhere the wind knocks me back down.

I need to create my story and write a brand new script for my life, one that involves me trusting myself, my own perceptions and judgments, and finding a way to crash through the walls I have built around myself for so long. I am excited, but I also find myself deep in an ocean of tears at unexpected moments.

"You're grieving," Dr. Stone says.

Yes, I know I have a lot to grieve, so he must be right, but the feelings have been buried alive, gasping for air, and clawing to get out. The words I need to talk about them, to give them breath support, are stuck so deep inside that I could barely utter the sounds much less articulate my thoughts even with him until now. I am on trauma overload.

In September, just a few weeks after I am discharged from Walter Reed, Steve and I have our legal separation hearing at the Rockville courthouse. He shows up with his lawyer, a big smile, and a bouquet of flowers. I stare at him in disbelief. What the hell is this? I take the flowers and then throw them back at him, telling him where he can put them.

On the witness stand, under oath, Steve freely admits to living with another woman and her two children. After all, what's the problem with that? I'm sure he thinks it is his right, because we are separated which in his mind frees him to do whatever he wants while the kids remain all my responsibility. He acts oblivious to the negative legal perception he is creating about himself, given the awful circumstances our family has faced. I see the shock and then a smirk on the judge's face, and the barely contained anger on Steve's lawyer's face. I can only imagine the conversations they will have after this hearing.

I have always known Steve to be a very intelligent person so I know it is not stupidity that makes him do and say these things. Despite our differences I begin to feel pity for him, for his confusion about what matters in life. When it is my turn to testify I hobble to the stand, swear in, and answer the questions my lawyer asks about Jeff's severe brain injury and my recent surgery for ovarian cancer.

My attorney has an easy job because I am a model witness, and I have a story that makes me look like a saint and Steve a jerk. I know I've won the case after my testimony winds up and the judge says to me, in a soft and sympathetic tone, "You can step down now, honey."

The court order arrives in the mail a few days later. Steve is ordered to pay small amounts of child support and alimony, and to make the mortgage payments on the house so that the boys and

I can stay there for at least two more years. I am given temporary full custody of Jeff and Travis and we set up a visitation schedule for Steve to have them with him every other weekend provided he has his girlfriend and her children leave the apartment.

Shortly before our separation hearing Steve and I went to court with Jeff for the follow-up hearing from his arrest. The case was dismissed because the judge understood about brain injury; it turns out he has a nephew who also has a TBI so he knew the memory problem we said Jeff has are quite real. Legally, Jeff is not able now to testify on his own behalf because he has what's called retrograde amnesia and cannot remember much what of happened the year before his TBI.

Steve and I are at least talking again, and working together better than we did over the summer. He even tries at times to apologize to me for the things he's done, but it isn't long before he stops paying his child support or alimony, and begins to appear at our house whenever he feels like it to see Jeff and Travis. My life is constant chaos and I tell him I cannot cope with him rearranging the schedule to suit himself and his girlfriend.

"You have to follow the court-ordered schedule if you want to see them," I tell him one night when he shows up unexpectedly. The kids are out with friends, so I stand at the front door refusing to let him in. "I can't have you just coming here whenever you want to and expecting us to accommodate you," I announce.

He looks down at me as if I am being completely unfair to him, because after all he has a complicated life with Cynthia and her kids. The old me would have been more sympathetic to his problems following the visitation schedule and would have accommodated him. But she is dead, may she rest in peace and never return.

"I'll have to get back to you on that," he says, although it's a long time before we hear from him again.

Steve stops making any of the payments he was ordered to make, so I am left with no income and little choice but to begin using up the little bit of savings I have. The scariest part is that I begin receiving notices of foreclosure on the house and threats to cut off our utilities. When I try to talk to my lawyer about it he doesn't return my calls, and then when he does he keeps advising me to "wait." He says we could charge Steve with Contempt of Court but he thinks it is a better strategy to let him get into arrearages and use it against him later. I tell him that will not help me if the kids and I are out on the streets, and he just laughs as if that was not a possibility. I begin to think I should find another lawyer but when I call a few they all want a retainer I can't afford.

I have weekly appointments at the oncology clinic at the Washington Hospital Cancer Institute and the numbers from my blood tests indicate that my health is improving. But I hate sitting with people who look like they are dying as we all wait for our names to be called, and I feel guilty because I know I am not as bad off as they are. Intellectually, I know I had cancer, and that I have lost my female reproductive organs, but it doesn't feel real to me. What I do feel is weak and tired all of the time, and I am sleeping too much.

To keep myself hopeful I focus on creating a new and better life, and I post written goals for myself on my bedroom wall near the door I walk past every day. Every morning I promise myself that I will do what is on that list to keep the promise I made to God when I was in the hospital. It doesn't matter if there is a God or not; it is really a promise from me to me.

The lyrics of a popular song called Break My Stride by Matthew Wilder say: "Nobody's gonna break my stride; I gotta keep on movin'..." That song is my mantra because I need to keep moving or I will surely die.

My new goals are simple but seem enormous: (1) find a new job that will give me time to work on my dissertation; (2) help Jeff so he can have a normal life someday; (3) get Travis through high school and off to college; and (4) get divorced as soon as possible.

I also hope to find a new someone to love but not necessarily marry. I'm not sure I ever want to get married again, but I do not want to be lonely and I am.

I had one of my visions the other day. I was in the kitchen and I looked over at the family room and saw a man, who wasn't really there, sitting on the sofa. There was also a young child playing on the floor in front of him. I could only see the back of his head so I don't know what he looked like and maybe that's good because I'm afraid I'm just crazy enough to go looking for him. I know it was silly, especially because I can't have any more children, but for a moment I felt a sense of peace and happiness and I enjoyed that. I'm not really looking for a new husband though.

My friend Judy is that friend everyone needs when getting divorced. The one you can talk to about your deepest feelings, even when it's a day you want to kill your ex, and then go out together to get drunk or maybe pick up men in a bar. She is my best misery-loves-company friend. We have a theory that a single woman should have about five men at a time; the Mormons have it backward. There should be one guy with plenty of money to take you out to expensive places and buy you gifts; one to fix things around the house; one to fix your car; one who is sensitive and a good listener; and one who is very sexy looking and terrific in bed. How could any one man meet all of our criteria?

I don't have the energy to go out much but when I can I jump at the chance to escape from the pain of my life. Dr. Stone keeps saying I am in denial about my hysterectomy and the fact that I can't have any more children, but I disagree.

"I had another dream about a baby," I tell him. "This one was crying, abandoned on the front porch, and when I walked out she held up her arms to me and said, "Help me!'"

"What do you think that's about?" he asks.

"Maybe it's about Jeff, or my dissertation, I don't know."

We toss around theories. Maybe the baby represented me because

I had abandoned parts of myself for so long. For whatever reason, I keep on having dreams about babies and it bothers me.

"Do you think it's because you can't have a baby anymore?" he asks.

Since he keeps going back to his denial theory, I figure it's obvious that it's his explanation and he wants me to say it was my idea.

I try to turn it around on him. "I don't think so, but do you?"

He never gives me the answers, just the questions. It drives me a little crazy at times, but I have to admit I do not know how I feel about losing this baby-making ability, this pre-ordained purpose of life for women that I was raised to believe in. I don't see why I would be grieving over that when I have two children already and don't want more. Yes, there was a time, earlier in my life, when I wanted to have a third child, just not with Steve. And then as I got close to forty I began thinking I was too old anyway. And I have a lot of other things to do, and certain things I was reluctant to admit, even to Dr. Stone.

A few months earlier, for instance, I met a nice guy named Pete, who seemed honest for a change. He was interesting to talk to and he came from a wealthy family, drove a Mercedes, and even took me flying in his airplane; what a fun adventure that was. I convinced myself I loved him, and I did in a way. Mainly because he was sympathetic about Jeff and said Steve was a fool. And he was honest; did I mention that? Honesty was something I thought men might be incapable of and it endeared him to me.

"You should marry him," Travis said with dollar signs in his eyes. Jeff agreed. But Pete and I had different politics and different goals in life, and he wanted to have a child.

Alas, sorry Travis, but it wasn't meant to be.

"I'm worried because I know I could fall in love with you but I can't," Pete said one night. I asked him what he meant.

"I have a trust fund and I want to have a child to leave it to. It's important, you know, for my family legacy."

A trust fund? Family legacy? He said he was from "old money" and I replied, "What's that? I'm from no money, so don't know the difference." He explained what old money meant to him. He said people from old money kept the old, worn family sofa (probably an expensive antique), and new money people threw old furniture out and got the expensive new stuff. Well, okay! I kept old furniture, even when the dog peed on it and I had to wash that spot out and it faded but still smelled. Did that make me like someone from old money? He didn't see the humor when I said that.

So after that conversation Pete and I both knew we didn't really have that much in common but I was still hurt that he didn't want to get involved with me because I couldn't have children anymore. We moved our relationship to being just friends, and for the first time I began to wonder how many other men would feel like Pete did about me not being able to have a baby. Was I defective now?

I put my guard back up and decided to be careful about letting anyone into my life once Steve and I were divorced. I would just date for fun and maybe sex. For a few months I went out on a lot of first dates and turned men down for anything more than that. There was a man named Kumar from India, who kept asking me out. Kumar was well educated, handsome, and had a high-level government job, but as we talked I learned that he was still living with his wife even though he said he was separated and getting a divorce.

"It was an arranged marriage, and we are not compatible," he said on the phone one day. So that made it okay?

"I have to think about this," I told him.

I would talk to Dr. Stone about it at my next appointment.

So, here I am, back in Dr. Stone's office, romantic confessions complete.

"Let me get this straight," he says in the slow and pointed manner that he uses when trying to tell me to pay attention because this is something important. "You are thinking of going out with another man you already know has lied to you?"

Okay, I get it. After spending the rest of the session analyzing this problem I see that I trust the wrong men. I have to admit it is possible that I only get involved with men who lie to keep myself from being open to a real relationship like the one I said I wanted. Ouch. Am I really doing this to myself? I'm not just the victim, but also my own perpetrator?

"Let's look at why," Dr. Stone suggests, launching a long journey into some parts of my past that I have avoided thinking about for my entire life.

"Maybe it is me who's afraid of intimacy," I admit to Dr. Stone the next time I see him. Of course he already knows that and I can almost hear him chuckle in his head even though he doesn't do it out loud. He just nods.

"Why do you think that is?" he asks.

I begin to see that I have chosen men who have all sorts of barriers to emotional intimacy. It is hard to accept that I might be creating my own relationship nightmares and that I am afraid of intimacy and commitment even though I say that's what I want. I have to work on why in order to change that. I decide to stop dating for the foreseeable future, until I get this fear of intimacy figured out. Any relationship I have in the future has to be different.

I also know that I still have a lot of real-life, present-day problems to resolve and dating might just be a means of avoiding that. I have no money to live on, no job, no divorce even. Jeff is a cognitively impaired young man who acts completely unpredictably and bizarrely at times; Travis rebels by staying out late or all night on the weekends. I am also back to eating too much junk and gaining weight again, a lifelong problem that I never can seem to get under control.

And then Christmas is upon us. Christmas is a day I just want to skip but I feel I have to do something. Instead of putting up a tree, I string lights around a big potted rubber tree plant and along the windows in the family room. I like it. Maybe I have a new holiday tradition now? It is festive and different, and it cheers me up to do something so non-traditional.

The holidays, however, are sad. The day after Christmas, 1989, I write in my journal:

> *It wasn't a great Christmas but it could've been a lot worse. At least Jeff is alive, the court ruling was in my favor, the kids are both with me, and I have friends even though they are all out of town for the holidays. Travis had a cold so we all just watched TV, ate junk food, and went to bed early on Christmas Eve. Travis gave me perfume and Jeff gave me house shoes. Steve called Christmas night and said he was out of the state and would not tell the kids where he was.*

Steve is just acting weirder and weirder, and I decide he must be having some sort of breakdown, but there isn't much I can do when he won't talk to me.

On New Year's Eve I try to focus on celebrating that 1989, the Year from Hell, is ending. A few good things help, too, like finding out Jeff had completed his one remaining high school English class and will be able to graduate in May at the Kennedy Center in DC. I am happy to be alive and not dying of cancer, and I try my best to remain hopeful that things for all of us will improve in 1990. The days of thinking I wanted to run away or die are gone. That all by itself is something to celebrate.

For my New Year's resolutions, which I make every year and usually accomplish (except for the one about losing weight) I expand and refocus my earlier list of goals to: (a) finish my dissertation proposal, (b) get my divorce finalized, (c) sell the house, (d) move to a new place of my own, and (e) find a good job where I could use my Ph.D. coursework to do something important, whatever that might be.

I still nurture the budding hope that Jeff will someday be able to support himself and go on to a normal adult life. He's still talking about going to college and I feel guilty for thinking of it selfishly, but having Jeff away would solve a lot of problems for me. I need a break, and maybe then I could pay more attention to Travis and start working on my dissertation.

I also find out, through Jeff's day treatment program, that the Maryland Department of Rehabilitative Services (DORS) will provide full financial support, including room and board, if Jeff goes to a four year college. They require that he take at least three classes, technically a full load of courses, and maintain a B average. Can he manage that? I'm not sure.

The financial burdens and worries are overwhelming; there are weeks I can't even afford to buy food for all of us. At those times we eat a lot of peanut butter and I become creative at fixing whatever we have in the cabinets.

I have been clinging to the hope that any day my lawyer would do something to make Steve honor his commitments and the court orders, but as time goes by, I only get a check every few months when Steve feels like it. I still have my small contract with Gallaudet which I use along with the once-in-awhile child support payments to pay bills, buy food, and put gas in the car. And I am so fortunate that my psychiatrist has waived his copayments until I have the money to pay him. But I hate living like this. There is just not enough money and the threats of utilities being cut off or the house going into foreclosure form a dark, ominous cloud on the horizon.

The only solution I can see is to finish my degree and get a good job. I want to be able to support us without Steve's help. Maybe I can do that with Jeff out of the house, so despite my worries I begin to see the possibility that it would be a good idea for Jeff to go away to college. Maybe doing something normal for his age will help him with his recovery too.

Jeff and I visit the various colleges and universities within a reasonable distance that have a good reputation for support services for students with disabilities, and we both get excited. When we talk about it he says all the right things to convince me that he knows what he needs to do to make this work. He promises he will get plenty of rest, use his memory aids, work with disability services to line up note-takers, and meet regularly with counselors on campus.

But I wonder: does he really understand that he needs to do all of that, or is he just saying it to sell me on the idea? I am learning that someone with a brain injury can be good at looking normal even when he isn't. I don't know if college is a good idea at all, but Jeff says he has goals to major in either psychology or education and I want to help him with that. I was always a parent who pushed my kids to learn new things and to set goals for themselves, and I'm just glad that in spite of his brain injury Jeff still has some ideas for his future.

I also know Jeff had always been a highly intelligent kid who scored high on the SAT and was in all advanced classes in high school. That was before his TBI, though. I don't know if he can manage the coursework, or being away from home and living in a university dorm where there will be so many distractions, or if he will even be able to find his way around to get to his classes. He gets lost taking the bus or metro anywhere and when he gets lost or confused he can get so angry at himself that it scares me.

Jeff's job coach, Bob, is a nice young man with his outpatient rehabilitation program who seems to understand Jeff pretty well so I talk to him about college choices, and he suggests his own alma matter, Indiana University of Pennsylvania (IUP) near Pittsburgh. It's a four-hour drive to the university through the western part of Pennsylvania and when we get there Jeff says he loves it. They offer good disability supports and the campus is small enough to be manageable but large enough to offer a variety of activities and academic programs.

I'm in so far over my head, guiding a nineteen-year-old brain-injured young man into adulthood and deciding whether he's ready to go away to school. I get conflicting advice from Bob who says he thinks Jeff would be fine, versus his neuropsychologist who suggests we wait a year. I obsess over the questions: What if I let him go away to school and something awful happens to him? Or, on the other hand, what if I hold him back by being so overprotective that he never gets to have a life? After all the pain and suffering he has been through, I just want to do the right thing by Jeff. So we send applications in to four universities and wait to see if he will be accepted.

SECTION II

*"Life isn't about waiting for the storm to pass.
It's about learning to dance in the rain."*

—Vivian Greene

*Following my release from Bryn Mawr
Rehabilitation Hospital of Malvern, PA into the
world of outpatient rehabilitation, I had another
important task to deal with: getting my education. I
do not have clear memories of the beginning of this
but I am aware that I spent a great deal of time in
the Counseling and Advising Building finding out
what class I had next, what time it started, and how
to get to it. I also remember being shocked by the
number of students who seemed to me to be milling
around the campus as I held my campus map in one
hand, my schedule in another with a finger locked
onto my current destination, and tried to make it
from one building to the next.*

—Jeff Bouck, TBI Survivor

Chapter 5

Dancing with Ed

I LOVE TO DANCE BUT WAS NEVER that talented; if I had received such a gift I might have wanted to be a professional dancer. Or singer, another gift I did not get. That's another future that did not select me, but I can still enjoy escaping into the feeling of moving to music and singing in the shower. After our horrible year in 1989, Jeff, Travis, and I were all ready to begin living and for me that meant going out dancing again.

On April 7, 1990 I celebrated my forty-second birthday by turning down a date with someone I knew was not right for me and went with my friend Judy and her new boyfriend to a Saturday night singles dance at the Washington Ethical Society. Judy and I were sitting away from the dance floor talking while the DJ played the usual oldies songs, when a guy I recognized from a similar singles dance called Discovery approached us. He sported a big smile and that determined "I'm going to dance with you!" look on his face. He was staring right at me.

"Oh, it's that guy Ed again," I said to Judy.

"He's not so bad," she said. Judy was in a new pro-men phase, trying to encourage me to date again because she was in love.

"No but he's just sort of average, and he's too friendly," I whispered.

I knew how silly that sounded but I also knew she would understand what I meant.

Friendly men scare me. I remember one poor sweet boy who kept pestering me to dance at a party in sixth grade and finally I punched him in the stomach. He never asked again, and if I knew where he was I'd apologize but I just hope he wasn't scarred permanently by me and my fear of boys at that age.

Ed looked like a persistent guy who would not take no for an answer and I guessed he wouldn't just dance with me once and leave me alone. I was right. He kept me dancing with him, telling me silly jokes and making funny comments about the songs or the people around us, and I was entertained so I didn't walk away.

Finally, I started to relax and enjoyed his company and yet some of his conversation was so goofy I felt a need to tell him. Maybe he'd leave me alone if I was blunt. I had learned a lot during my years of separation from Steve and dating, and I knew how to be just rude enough to make someone go away. My natural tendency to be friendly and sensitive to feelings was easy to put aside if I felt threatened.

"You're weird," I said as we danced to a slow song. I didn't care if he left me standing there, and I was proud of myself because I was getting really good at being direct with men, probably because I felt I had nothing to lose and didn't want a man in my life. It helped to not care so much like I did when I first met Steve. Separation and divorce does that to a lot of women I've observed.

"Yes, I resemble that remark," he said with a laugh. Nothing fazed this guy. "I have been told that before."

His genuine smile and warm blue eyes drew me to him in spite of myself and I had an unfamiliar stab of guilt about insulting him. I usually didn't care about the feelings of these men I met who all seemed predatory, until I got to know one of them at least. So, I wondered, why now and why him? Maybe I should give him a chance? I began to relax, the cheap wine making me lean more toward flirting than pushing him away.

"You're weird, but kind of cute," I said with a smile, and as he smiled back he kissed me lightly on the lips. At that moment the DJ announced that they had a special song to play for Janis, and the old song "Happy Birthday Sweet Sixteen" filled the room. Ed looked at me in surprise.

"It's your birthday?" he asked. I nodded, embarrassed to be singled out in the crowd but pleased that my friends remembered.

"Happy birthday!" he said, giving me a hug that felt so sincere I couldn't help but hug him back. He was keeping my attention now and I settled into staying with him instead of running to the restroom like I sometimes did when a man got too close.

Ed was different from my usual type; he was not the tall handsome one who stood by himself in the corner drinking a beer and not talking. The guy I usually zoomed in on, and tried to get through his shell thinking that he needed me. No wonder I ended up unhappy and lonely.

I reminded myself that Dr. Stone and I had agreed just the week before that I needed to be open to someone different, someone like Ed who seemed to want to communicate and have fun. So I kept dancing with him the rest of the evening and in between dances I learned more about him because, unlike the other men I knew, he talked incessantly. I found out that he was an Information Technology manager with the District of Columbia public schools, and I told him I was a Ph.D. student at Gallaudet University.

"Hey, I've been there!" he said. "My computer job is my day job, but I also umpire baseball and referee basketball, and I've officiated their games a few times. Did you know the football huddle was invented at Gallaudet?" he asked. I could tell he wanted to impress me so I played along.

"No I didn't know that but it makes sense," I said. "Do you know sign language?"

Looking proud he said, "I know a few signs, like for colors so I can call out the teams by their colors when I need to." He showed me what he knew for a few of the colors. When he signed "white," moving his hand up and down in front of his chest, I couldn't help but laugh.

"That's not white," I told him. "That's the sign for horny." He turned red and laughed.

I showed him the correct sign for white and he practiced it with me. "They've probably been having a good time talking about me while I made a fool of myself," he said still laughing. This guy was funny! He made me smile, something I had not done much of for about a year and had missed.

I laughed out loud when the DJ played the oldies song "Shout," and Ed, dressed in a nice suit, threw himself down on the floor in front of me and did the old dance called the alligator. Out of the corner of my eye I saw Judy and her boyfriend smiling and watching us.

I have always been the extroverted type of person who is the last to leave a party, and so I stayed to help clean up at the end of the evening. Before he left, Ed found me and asked for my phone number. I gave it to him. I figured I'd go out with him once or twice, if he even called, just for fun. He did call the next day and we had a good chat, again a rather silly conversation, and we made a date for two weeks later because we were both busy the next weekend.

For our first date Ed picked me up at the house and we went to a concert at Georgetown University to hear a popular rock group called the Kinks, and then we went out for dessert afterward. We talked all evening and I got to know him as someone with more depth than I had given him credit for. When he brought me home we sat on the sofa making out like teenagers and I knew I would be going out with Ed more than just a few times.

After our third date he showed up at my house in his umpire's shirt and pants and said he had just finished a baseball game in our neighborhood so he thought he'd come by to talk. I made him a sandwich and then we settled into my living room sofa. I wondered what was so urgent and important that he didn't just call, but I was glad to see him.

"I feel like this is going too fast and I'm getting scared because my relationships in the past have not worked out," he said. "I want to tell you everything so if you are going to reject me you can do it now," he said. Barely taking a breath, he began telling me the story of his life.

He said that he had never been married, probably because of his quirks, and he wanted me to know about them. He had a long list from how he grew up with a father who was an abusive alcoholic and a mother who was a Holocaust survivor, to the present day and how he just seemed to always say or do the wrong things in relationships with women. He told me how lonely he had been and how afraid he was to approach women, something I would not have guessed the way he pursued me at the Ethical Society.

"I have seen you at Discovery and had a crush on you for a long time," he said.

Wow, I had never imagined someone would come to me, all on his own initiative, and do this. We sat there talking for four hours, the boys coming and going and grinning at us, and I listened as he explained a lot of things about his life, what he was doing to work on himself, and what he was looking for in a relationship. It matched what I wanted.

"I think I'm a diamond in the rough, and I just need someone to teach me," he said at last. And he paused to stare at me as if he expected some kind of negative response.

Uh-oh, this was scary. He wants a teacher about relationships? I was the woman who read every self-help relationship book published, and had spent years analyzing my relationship problems with Steve. That had my name all over it! And what made it worse was that he would be so vulnerable and honest with me so soon. Everything he said spelled long-term relationship and emotional intimacy and I was suddenly afraid I was starting to fall in love. The protective barriers I had put up around myself, like the walls of a fortress, were coming down and I began to shiver even though it was a warm day.

"There's something else I need to tell you. You may have noticed something different about me," he said watching my eyes intently. I had noticed; of course I had. He was not very coordinated and he was fidgety, constantly touching his face or gesturing when he talked. I thought for a minute before answering.

"Yes, I thought maybe some kind of learning disability, hyperactivity?"

"Cerebral Palsy," he said, and then it all made sense. "I was born with mild CP, and didn't walk until I was almost four years old. My mother carried me and...." He paused, looking scared that he had told me so much. I interrupted him with a kiss.

"You don't know what I do for a living, do you?" I asked. He shook his head and I went on. "I'm a speech pathologist and I've worked with a lot of people with CP and other disabilities, so it's fine. I understand now." We both cried a little. It seemed that the pieces of our lives fit together like a jigsaw puzzle in ways I would never have expected from someone I had met at a singles' dance. We decided sometimes relationships like ours just happen when you least expect it.

I worried that I would not be able to set limits with him, but I loved that he was telling me these things about himself without me even having to ask. As we kept talking I told him more and more about my life and my fears, and I even took a leap of faith and told him what worried me about him.

"I'm afraid that you're the kind of guy who will try to make me into your mother and then resent me for it," I said. I had developed a tendency to be direct about my observations; some men liked it and some ran for the hills. Ed didn't run and just nodded instead.

"If I do that just tell me," he said. "I don't ever want anyone to take care of me the way mother did. It made me feel I could never be independent and I hated that."

We discussed it and agreed that the most important thing to both of us was to keep our support systems in place and, yes, he was in therapy like me. He was That Guy, the one I had been wishing for, the one who was all screwed up but knew it and was in therapy. The one who I didn't think existed and had given up on. We decided we needed time together, time apart, and time with friends and that it was important to talk things over.

Ed made no effort to control me or argue with anything I said I was looking for, even when I told him I was not ready for a committed relationship. He said he hoped I would change my mind and that he was going to date only me. I was still not sure I was capable of being in a serious relationship and I tucked away a small fear that I might ruin this thing with Ed eventually.

Then he said he wanted someone to travel with him because he loved to go on trips and had always had to do that alone. That scared me even more because I had never had that with Steve except for visiting family or traveling some when we were stationed in Europe. How could I leave my kids and all of my problems to go off on a vacation? But I told him I would think about it.

And so began my new life, the life I had wanted for so long, even though I did not know that's what was happening on the day Ed came to my house all sweaty from nervousness and umpiring. How could I have seen that he would make such a change in everything I knew?

I was trying to move on from tragedy to a better place of survival and joy, and so were my two sons. Jeff continued to push for more and more independence and so did Travis. It was their job to do that, to argue with me, and I now understood that it was my job to not cave in as I had in the past. After what had happened to Jeff I was becoming more of a parent now and less of a friend, which meant we had our ups and downs, but I knew it was progress. And in so many ways it was easier to make that change as a single parent than with a co-parent who did not back me up.

Ed was over-the-top excited about our new relationship and wanted me to meet everyone he knew at work, his relatives in Pennsylvania, and even his therapist. I said no to meeting his therapist but went with him to meet his relatives and introduced him to a few people I knew. I felt a need to keep the brakes on because he obviously wasn't going to. It was new behavior for me to hold back and be the more reserved person in a relationship, and I kind of liked it. Instead of me doing what I used to do with men, I tried to do nothing and left it up to him and he did all the right things. He called me to talk almost every night and asked me how I felt about life and what I wanted.

"Ed, what's the most important thing in life?" I asked him once. I liked to cut to the chase.

"Being useful," he said without hesitation. "What about you?"

Ed always asked me how I felt about anything, and I was not used to that. I was a lonely woman who had been screaming in the middle of a dark forest with no one to listen.

"Self-expression," I said. Not only did he accept that, and seemed to like it, but he wanted to know more about how I felt and why that was important to me. This was an entirely foreign type of man to me, one who wanted to get to know me and let me know him as completely as I had always wanted someone to allow.

My friends asked me why I wanted to date someone who had never been married before. They said there must be a lot wrong with him!

"Well, for one thing he knows how to be single, he has his own house, he can cook, and I love it that he has no ex-wife or children," I told them. "And he tries really hard to make this work."

It was impossible to explain to anyone how much it meant to me that Ed worked so hard on our relationship after years of me trying to make my marriage to Steve work and feeling that he would not even meet me halfway. Ed also got along with my kids which was very important to me after all they had been through the previous few years.

When Ed first met Jeff, he held out his hand and said, "Hi, I'm Ed."

Jeff smiled his still lopsided grin, and said, "Hello, I'm God!"

Silly speech did not bother Ed at all; he was pretty silly himself. He just laughed and shook hands with Jeff, and that mattered to me more than I could say at the time. Other men I had been out with didn't say it but I could sense that they were uncomfortable with Jeff and his brain injury, and with all of the problems I had.

Ed wasn't scared off by my crazy life and in fact he said it meant a lot to him. He thought he could be good for Jeff because he understood what it was like to have a disability people were confused by. He wanted to help my son through his brain injury recovery and to help Jeff gain some independence; how could I not love someone like that? Not only did he love me, but he wanted to help Jeff?

Travis was harder. He wasn't convinced about Ed. Ed didn't fit the mold of what he thought I should have if I married again and Ed sensed Travis's skepticism.

"I don't know what to do for Travis," he said one night. "I don't know how to relate to him. How can I help him?"

"You can't," I said. "Travis has a lot of pride and he doesn't want a substitute father, but I think he needs to feel less responsible for things because he's so young and had so much on him. So maybe you could just give him money once in a while so he doesn't feel it's all up to him." At age sixteen Travis worked and went to school and paid for his own expenses because I couldn't. So that's what Ed tried to do without going overboard and I watched with relief as Travis gradually began to accept him. Ed thought it helped that Travis's friends who played baseball knew him because he was an umpire, and maybe it did.

Ed and I began to see each other every weekend and talk on the phone during the week. One night we were at his house and I started to shake as he kissed me.

"What's wrong?" he whispered in my ear, holding me tightly.

"I'm afraid of falling in love with you," I said. It felt as if I was physically letting go of something inside, and I had the sense of tumbling down into a deep well. It was a feeling of completely losing control that I had never experienced before and my head said I should not let this happen but my heart just gave in.

"It's too late for me," he said.

After meeting Ed, I never did date anyone else and the commitment I had previously been afraid would be too hard for me came easily. He filled up my life with concerts, dinners out, and sleepovers at his house or mine, and he met my emotional needs with love and the sense of closeness I had been craving. I was never lonely with Ed even when we were not together; I always felt him with me and he called me a lot and told me what he was doing and where he was even when I didn't ask.

He even got excited about taking me grocery shopping and I hated grocery shopping after so many years of doing it all and standing in line at Army commissaries. This was an unexpected bonus!

One Friday night about two months after we began seeing each other we were together at my house and he said, "Whatcha want to do?"

"I don't know. What do you want to do?" We were getting into more of the hanging out, less planned evenings.

"You want to go grocery shopping?" he asked with a look of hopefulness. I stared at him in disbelief. "I'll buy you groceries and carry your bags!" he said. Was I dreaming? All of my determination to keep my options open just faded away and by the summer of 1990 we were a couple.

There were times, however, when I questioned our relationship. I told him I thought we were from different cultures. He was from that foreign land of the never-married, living like a big kid, and I was from the country of overly-responsible-married-with-children. I felt like sometimes we spoke a different language. But we bridged that cultural gap and began to build a real relationship based on trust, good communication, and shared values. I felt emotionally safe with Ed in a way I never had with anyone else.

The only problem was that with our different lifestyles we had vastly different ideas about fun and adventure, and we had very different levels of energy. When he asked me to go to Hawaii with him I panicked. I didn't see how I could leave Jeff and Travis alone for a week.

"They'll be fine," he said. "Jeff's nineteen years old and Travis is seventeen. It's time to let go."

Let go? What was he talking about? We argued and I told him he didn't understand because he never had children, never saw his child lying inert in a coma, never watched his marriage fall apart, never had cancer and feared dying and leaving broken teenagers on their own. He said I was smothering my kids like his mother had done with him.

Here it was at last: proof that we were not compatible. I wanted to go with him to all the places he kept talking to me about, places I had never seen, but I was afraid and he just did not understand. It was, to me, as if Ed was a child with no parenting responsibilities while I had always felt the weight of putting my kids first.

"You don't see that you deserve a vacation," he said. "Vacations help us to gain a new perspective on things, to be happier." I thought of a vacation without my kids as frivolous and irresponsible and he was telling me it was a spiritual enrichment?

"I can't pay for anything," I told him in an effort to put a stop to his pressure. He probably knew that, since I never had money for anything, but I wanted to make it clear.

"Don't worry, it's my treat," he said. What could I say after that?

"Go," the kids told me when I discussed it with them. "We can manage here just fine."

As we flew to California and on to the beautiful island of Kauai, a long way from my sons in Maryland, I was wracked with guilt and worry. Having fun like this, feeling free, allowing myself to go on a romantic getaway, was not me at all.

Who was this person I was becoming? Selfish like my father had told me I was? What if something happened to Jeff or Travis, like the day I was on an airplane about to leave and Jeff was in that accident? I was still obsessing over my fears about the kids when we got off the plane and were greeted by women in hula skirts who hung beautiful flowered leis around my neck. Ed was beaming with pride that he had made those arrangements for me.

In Kauai we stayed at a beautiful hotel near the beach and watched the most gorgeous sunsets I had ever seen. We hiked though a rainforest, watched Hawaiian dancers, and took a boat tour along the incredible Na Pali coastline. I had never had that kind of experience before, just being a tourist and doing things purely for fun. With Steve there were always so many financial problems that the only vacations we took, except for a few while we lived in Europe, were to visit our parents or camp out for a weekend with the kids and dog.

I tried to let myself enjoy the trip but the contrast between the luxury of vacation and the realities of my life back in Maryland were overwhelming and made it hard for me to relax as much as Ed wanted me to, and I felt additional guilt over that. I could tell he was disappointed at those times.

One afternoon we were taking a nap and I got a phone call from Travis.

"Mom!" he said. "Jeff is running up a hundred dollar bill at Blockbusters!"

Jeff had apparently been renting movies on our account and forgetting to take them back so we now owed a hundred dollars or more, and Travis was understandably angry with him for wasting that money when we had so little.

"There's not much I can do here in Hawaii, is there?" I said. I talked to Jeff and he was confused about where he had put the movies or how many he had rented. All I could do was tell him not to rent any more movies. I was upset but Ed laughed about it.

"If that's the worst thing that happens, it's fine," he said. "See? They're okay." He had the positive perspective of someone who had not experienced trauma, that feeling of safety and security that I lost when Jeff had his TBI and a black cloud descended on my life. I could never again feel secure that little things were not big things when it came to my kids. What if that small irresponsible behavior of Jeff's was only a precursor to doing something worse, and then I would get a call that one or both of them had been in a car accident or had set the house on fire?

Three days into the trip I began vomiting and having intense stomach pain, and I assumed it was because of my anxiety about leaving my kids alone. Or maybe the gods were punishing me for being so selfish and running away from my responsibilities. Ed said I was probably sick from eating too much at the hotel luau the night before, and I had to admit that could be true since we did overindulge in fatty pork and too many desserts.

My secret fear was that I had cancer again. The truth was that I had been sick like this off and on but had not told Ed or anyone else. It started when Jeff was at Bryn Mawr and I was in Malvern for the weekend. I spent many evenings after visiting him throwing up in the bathroom of my hotel room but I assumed it was from the stress and all the junk food I was eating. Later, after my hysterectomy, I thought it must have been the cancer and surgery. It seemed to come over me in bouts every week or so, and sometimes I was so sick I could barely eat for a day or two. The pain was unbearable.

I came home from that trip and went to bed, but the stabbing pain in my stomach and side would not go away. The following day I told Ed on the phone how sick I was and he dismissed it and said I was exaggerating. We didn't talk until the next day when he called to apologize and see how I was. I told him again that I was in pretty bad shape and he said if I really was that sick I should go to the doctor which I knew but was resisting. With his urging, I finally crawled out of bed later in the morning and drove myself to Walter Reed and saw the same doctor who did my hysterectomy.

She took one look at me and asked, "Do you know you are jaundiced?" I shook my head. She told me to look in her office mirror and, sure enough the person staring back was a yellow version of me.

"I'm admitting you right now," she said giving the nurse some papers to take to the medical unit of the hospital.

I had gall bladder disease and it had begun to affect my liver. I could not go home. Once again there I was back at Walter Reed, though this time I hoped I had someone to help.

I called the kids to tell them, and then I called Ed and asked him to check on Jeff and Travis and make sure they were okay because I was in the hospital. He sounded shocked but said he would give them a call. Over the next few days my friends and my kids came to visit, but no Ed. I waited and waited, and then we had a huge fight on the phone when Ed said he didn't know what to do. That made no sense to me. I was in the hospital and he didn't know what to do?

I told Judy about it when she came to visit. "I may have to break up with him," I said. "He's not who I thought he was."

She nodded and agreed. Judy was logical about these things, and I needed that at the moment because I was a wreck and couldn't be sure I was thinking clearly. I loved Ed but I was not going to continue seeing someone who had so little compassion when I needed him. I had already been in that kind of relationship with Steve, so why would I stay involved with another man like that?

The next day when Ed still didn't show up or call, I decided we were finished and when he finally called I told him so. I was proud that I had changed. I was willing to stand up for myself at the expense of losing someone I loved, something I had never been able to do before. I told him how sick I was, that he was a really big disappointment to me, and I said, "Shape up or we are finished!" Then I hung up on him.

It felt good to be free of the desperate need to hang onto someone if he didn't treat me right, the glue that kept me stuck in a marriage like that for so many years. Even though I cried after that conversation with Ed, I knew I did the right thing.

Ed showed up the next day with balloons and flowers and endless apologies. He explained that he had been paralyzed by fear because his mother died of leukemia when he was nineteen. She died at Johns Hopkins at the end of Ed's freshman year away at college and he got to the hospital just in time to say goodbye. Having been a child with CP, and dependent on his mother more than most boys his age, he was rocked by losing her and knew he did not deal well with illness and hospitals.

"I'm so sorry, and I want to do better. Will you give me a chance?" he asked.

I never thought I'd meet a man who would admit he was wrong and be open about why he did what he did. Those men did not exist in the world I came from and my mother had always told me men were incapable of that kind of vulnerability in relationships so I never expected it. I decided to forgive him and give him the chance he wanted, but I did let him know I would not be okay if he did it again.

Because I had been so stubborn in refusing to get help when I first became sick, now the doctors had to pump me full of medications and vitamins to get me well enough to do the gall bladder surgery. I was in the hospital three weeks and got home just in time to help Travis get ready for his senior year of high school and Jeff ready to go away to college. It was a lot to take care of and once again I was weak, on pain medications, and unable to drive. But unlike the previous summer when I had my hysterectomy, I now had a partner who stayed with me to help. Ed made good on his promise to do better.

A few days after I was home from the hospital Ed, Jeff, and I packed up the car and we all headed west on I-70, with Ed driving my Honda Wagovan to take Jeff off to college. He was accepted everywhere he applied and we had selected the beautiful IUP in Pennsylvania which the Maryland DORS said they would pay for. Jeff said he was excited about their well-known programs in the two fields he was interested in, teaching and psychology. I was hopeful that their good support program for students with disabilities would make it possible for him to be successful his first year away at college and all the way through to earning a degree.

As we drove out of Montgomery County I could not help but reflect on how different this drive was from the last time, a little over a year before, when Steve and I moved Jeff to another place in Pennsylvania. This time Jeff was not going to a rehabilitation hospital but was actually going away to college! I couldn't believe how much life had changed in such a relatively short time and in ways I had not thought possible in March, 1989. It was another lesson in the series of lessons I was getting that the future was indeed unpredictable.

We stopped mid-morning for a coffee break in the small Pennsylvania town of Breezewood, and by noon we arrived at the campus of IUP with Jeff driving, sitting proudly in the driver's seat for the first time since his accident. I was lying in the backseat with my eyes shut, panicked that Ed was letting Jeff drive. I couldn't even watch, but Ed patiently talked Jeff through the busy intersections as we neared the university, giving him directions for each turn, helping him to negotiate the campus traffic and crowded streets. Ed just understood from his own history of struggling for independence how important it was to Jeff to arrive at college behind the wheel.

As we unloaded suitcases and put linens on the bed I saw my brain-injured, still very thin son looking around in joy, and I was glad we had made this decision. He had been through so much that damaged his self-esteem and I could see how happy he was to be going away to college like his friends. I knew he was probably thinking: hey, I'm back to normal!

Jeff was still easily fatigued so, as an accommodation for his TBI, I had arranged for him to have a single room with no roommate. That way he could sleep when he needed to and have a distraction free place to study. It was a small room with only a single bed, dresser, desk, chair, and closet but to Jeff I could tell it represented a new life in the same way that my decision to finally end my marriage did for me. I could relate to his excitement. To him that dorm room was his own place, a start to his independent adult life.

Before we left I reminded him that I had put a few hundred dollars in a checking account for him and we reviewed how to use the checkbook. I also reminded him to eat all of his meals in the cafeteria because it was covered by his room and board plan which DORS paid for along with the tuition. With very little money to give him, I felt bad because I was sure that I had not provided what other parents did, but he was happy. He couldn't wait, he said, to go to the cafeteria for lunch and start being a college student.

I didn't want to go and kept stalling, reminding him to do his laundry and check in with the counselors, until he finally said "Mom, I'll be okay," and gave me a hug. He wanted us to leave and so we did. I waited to break into sobs until Ed and I were alone at a nearby restaurant for lunch.

"I just don't know if this was the right decision. He's still so fragile, and what if something happens to him?" I said through my tears.

"No, you are doing the right thing," Ed said, holding my hand across the table. He was always so reassuring. I wanted to go back to the dorm and take Jeff home, but Ed talked me off the ledge and after lunch we drove home.

Over the next week Travis and I settled into a routine that was much less stressful with Jeff out of the house, and I began to relax and think this may have been the right decision after all. I could actually get things done without Jeff constantly talking to me or needing my help with something, or just wanting me to watch a movie on TV with him.

At the end of the first week the phone rang and it was Jeff.

"I'm homesick. Can you come get me? I want to come home," he said.

When I left home to attend IUP I was 25 years younger than I am now and so had MUCH less perspective than I currently do. Back then, I believed that despite whatever fears I may have, perhaps even BECAUSE of them, I could and would accomplish anything. I mean after all I HAD graduated high school, I HAD relearned to walk, I HAD learned what I believed to be every coping skill I would ever need to deal with my disability (TBI). I was good to go. Also, I was looking forward to finally having a place of my own. I was going to have a private dorm room. With everything I have mentioned above, plus my awareness that the academics of high school HAD always come naturally to me, I knew the upcoming year would be nothing but fun in the sun. Boy was that wrong.

—Jeff Bouck, TBI Survivor

Chapter 6

Jeff Meets an Italian Princess

HEARING JEFF SOUNDING SO LOST and lonely, saying he wanted to be home and missed us, I felt sick with regret.

"Jeff, what's wrong? Have you met the other guys in your dorm?" I asked.

"Not really," he said in a flat tone.

"Are your classes okay?"

"Yes."

"It's normal to get homesick at first," I said, trying to keep things light. "Maybe you could join a club on campus or find some way to make friends?"

I wanted so much to get in my car and drive immediately to IUP but I had read somewhere that it was to be expected that a college freshman would be homesick and that parents should not give in to it. It took my best acting skills to sound positive, and to try to make him feel better, and eventually he laughed and said he would stay and give it a try.

I did think it might be good to go pick him up and bring him home for a weekend, but I couldn't drive so soon after my surgery. For the next month we talked on the phone frequently and he stopped saying he was homesick.

At mid-term I got reports on his grades and they were surprisingly good, two As and a B. When we talked on the phone he also said he was meeting people.

"I have a girlfriend," he said.

"That's nice," I told him. "What's she like?"

"She's from Italy," he said. "Her name is Bertha."

I was pleased for him that he was connecting with people and looking forward to spending time with him over the Thanksgiving break. We talked about our plans to pick him up, and he asked if Bertha could come for a visit.

"Really? It's that serious?" I asked.

"We're engaged," he said. He referred to her as his fiancée, and I was taken aback and worried.

"Jeff, she's not your fiancée," I said, in an effort to bring him into reality. "But I do want to meet her."

Ed and I decided maybe the best thing was just to keep it all low key and wait to see what she was like over the Thanksgiving holiday. The day before Thanksgiving, Ed and I drove to IUP to pick Jeff up, assuming Bertha would be with him, but when we got there Jeff said she could not come after all. I was so happy to see him, and I didn't want to rock the boat by demanding to meet her, so we said maybe next time and headed home for the holidays.

On the four-hour drive back to our house we had time to ask a lot of questions and, as Jeff talked on and on about Bertha, Ed and I exchanged worried looks because his story made no sense. I asked him how they met, where her family lived, how old she was, things that any mother would ask about a new girlfriend she'd never met.

"She works at the arcade next to the dorm," he said.

"How did she end up here in Pennsylvania?" I assumed she was a student and working part-time.

"She's divorced and from Italy. Her father is a king there so she's a princess."

I tried to keep a straight face. Was he serious? Glancing at him in the rear view mirror, and judging from his tone of voice, he was perfectly serious and believed what he was saying.

"We're close to the same age but she's a little older, and she has a daughter," he explained.

What? A child? I was beginning to panic because this sounded like even more of a problem than I had realized.

"How old is her daughter?" I asked in alarm.

"I don't know but she's a teenager. Bertha was forced to marry young, like when she was about fourteen years old, and now she has a teenage daughter, maybe fifteen or sixteen years old. I'm not sure."

I tried to keep my cool but it was hard. "Jeff, there is no king in Italy so she's not an Italian princess. And if she got married at fourteen and had a child sixteen years ago, she would be at least thirty now. Something is just not right with her story, don't you see that?"

Jeff was always good at math, taking advanced calculus in high school, and yet he continued to insist she was about the same age as him and a princess.

"Jeff, think about it," I said, trying to stop myself from yelling at him. "She's an Italian princess living in rural Pennsylvania? Named Bertha? You really believe that?"

"Yes."

He got mad at me then and clammed up, saying he didn't want to talk about his fiancée with me. I knew then that Jeff was not playing with a full deck and I had to do something.

When we got home Ed and I talked in my bedroom. How could Jeff be doing so well in his classes and yet have such crazy lack of logic about this woman? How could he be so incapable of figuring this out?

The answer was as always simple: he had a brain injury. This was the part of life after traumatic brain injury that people doing research or presentations about TBI did not always understand; what made it all so difficult for everyone around the person with a TBI and for that person. From Jeff's perspective, I knew he honestly thought we were being unfair and unreasonable. For a young person without a brain injury there might be disagreement with parents about something, but reality would normally be in there somewhere and there could be a point of seeing each other's perspective. But Jeff's brain was telling him that this woman, whoever she was, was not lying to him and we were being unfair to her in suggesting she was. How could we problem-solve when we saw the situation so differently?

The answer was that we couldn't, but we kept trying. It was like arguing with a drunk person about why he should stop drinking while he was drunk and partying. Over Thanksgiving Jeff talked to this so-called fiancée on the phone, but when I tried to talk to her, she hung up. Ed tried to reason with Jeff and told him she was not who she said she was, and this might not be a healthy relationship.

"Jeff, why won't she talk to us or meet us?" he asked.

"She doesn't want to meet you guys because she knows you do not like her," he told us with an angry look.

Travis was furious with Jeff. "Dude, this is fucked up," he said. He also tried to use logic with Jeff but it went nowhere. The more we all talked about it, the more defensive Jeff became and Thanksgiving at our house that year was not at all peaceful or even thankful.

I scheduled an appointment for Jeff to see his neuropsychologist, hoping he could help Jeff to see reality. By the end of the Thanksgiving visit Jeff said that maybe he should end this relationship, and I relaxed a little. He was sounding much more normal and it would only be three weeks before he was home for Christmas break. What could happen in that short time? We drove him back to IUP at the end of Thanksgiving and tried to encourage him to focus on his classes and just spend time with other people, maybe ask another girl out on a date.

The next time we talked on the phone Jeff said he did not break up with Bertha and was back to believing her story and saying they were engaged. I told him this time, when we picked him up for the

Christmas break, we definitely had to meet her. He said that would be okay, but when we got there Jeff went to the arcade near his dormitory and came back alone saying she was not there and he didn't know where she was.

I got his first semester grades and was happy to see that Jeff passed all of his classes with a B average as DORS required. I was so proud of him for being able to do college level work not quite two years after being in a coma and an inpatient brain injury hospital. But we all argued throughout the winter break about Bertha until, once again, he said he could see that we were right and he needed to break up with her.

IN JANUARY JEFF BEGAN his second semester at IUP and right away I began to get calls from Steve and my father saying Jeff was calling them to borrow money. They both said he told them we would not give him any money for food and that he was hungry.

"He sounds crazy," my father told me. We had not been talking so he was even apologetic for calling, but I said I was glad he did.

"What's he saying?" I asked.

"He said he's getting married, and you won't help them."

"He's not engaged," I told him. "He's confused. So don't give him any money and please tell other family members not to give him money if he calls them. This is because of his brain injury."

"Well, he calls her his fiancée. And this isn't because of a brain injury. It's a matter of bad character and that's because of how he's been raised!"

As always, he made Jeff's problems, or anything going wrong in my life, my fault. I was trying to develop what Ed called a "shit shield" to my parents' verbal abuse and so I just thanked my father for calling and got off the phone.

Next I called Jeff to try to talk to him and he hung up on me. I called Steve to see what Jeff was telling him.

"He said that you're jealous of his fiancée."

Unlike my parents, Steve at least understood that Jeff was confused and that it was because of his TBI, and he was worried about him like we were. We talked for a long time and it just felt good to be able to share that role of co-parent again with him. He offered to do whatever he could to help and I told him I would let him know.

On Feb 23, 1991 I wrote in my journal:

> *I am so upset about Jeff. He called again yesterday and was so mad because he said I'm calling people and putting down his fiancée, and telling them not to give him money. He said he's going to get a protection from abuse order against me. She's getting him to apply for food stamps, disability, and encouraging him to write hot checks all over town.*

I continued to call Jeff and he finally did start talking to me again, but remained defensive and confused. Ed and I decided to just wait for him see the reality of what he was involved in, and for the relationship to end.

On March 5 my journal entry was:

> *Jeff went to the IUP police tonight, or they went out and found him, I'm not sure. They called me at 8:30 p.m. and said he'd requested he be voluntarily committed to a hospital. Travis was there holding my hand and feeling bad for Jeff too.*

Poor Jeff, my heart was breaking for him. After the police called me I drove, crying most of the way, to a truck stop on the highway in Pennsylvania where an officer met me with Jeff and his suitcase. He was so sympathetic to Jeff and to me, and said the other guys in the dorm had seen this woman around and they were worried about him. They finally called the police when Jeff didn't come back to his room for a few days and the police found a suicide note on his desk. They picked him up, walking alone on the edge of town, and took him to the hospital where he was evaluated. The doctors decided he was not a threat to himself or anyone else, but he was very confused and depressed and needed to come home.

Jeff said when he finally realized what was happening with Bertha he didn't know what to do. He didn't remember much, and couldn't explain what he did remember, but he said he was out on the highway that evening the police found him because he wanted a car to hit him.

Over the next few days I learned more from talking on the phone to the campus police. This woman, Bertha, had some very bad and dangerous accomplices, five aliases, and was getting Jeff to write hot checks and submit applications for disability with her as his guardian.

"The university will be filing charges against her," the officer said. "And you and your son will need to be there."

"I can't pay a lawyer," I told him.

"That's not necessary. I'll be there to represent you and tell what happened," he said.

We had a court hearing and the university provided me with a room for two days so that I could stay there at no charge. When Jeff and I walked into the courtroom I saw Bertha and her daughter for the first time and there was nothing Italian or princess-like about her. She was about the same age as me and very unattractive, and I could not imagine how Jeff could have seen her the way he did. It was shocking to realize, to fully comprehend, how damaged his perceptions were.

Jeff testified about what he believed to be true, which was sad but oddly perfect because it demonstrated to the judge that he was not in touch with the reality of the situation. I testified about his brain injury and confusion, and the so-called "fiancée" Bertha got on the stand and talked about how he had given her money and other things as a "gift between lovers." She was using the legal terminology to make it all legitimate and clearly knew what she was doing. She was a pro.

She was convicted of fraud. The judge said he was sympathetic to us but I did not have legal guardianship for Jeff so there was nothing to prevent him from being liable for the hot checks and other documents he had signed. Bertha was ordered to give him back some of the possessions she had taken from him, and we got a protection order to keep her away from him.

I took Jeff home and the university administrators granted him a temporary leave of absence from his classes. On the way out of town, after the hearing, I drove Jeff to each store where he had written bad checks and made him go in to explain, and pay them a little of the money he owed.

Over the next few months Steve and I paid Jeff's debts for him, and as always Jeff said all the right things when we discussed what had happened. He said he had learned a lot from the experience and could see that his judgment was still impaired. Did he really, though? Did he actually learn from this? I couldn't tell. But I knew that I had learned a lot.

I was rattled by seeing how serious Jeff's cognitive problems still were, and that they could be potentially life threatening. I had been wrong; he was not ready to handle the level of independence I had thought he could. And now he was home again, and I was not sure what to do next. My hopes for a new life were fading. This con artist relationship scared Ed too and for the first time he was angry with Jeff and began questioning whether he wanted to be involved with me and my little messed up family.

"I didn't understand before about the realities of Jeff's brain injury," he said when we argued about it one night. "I just don't know if I can do this."

On March 11, 1991 I wrote in my journal:

I think I'm realizing how scared I am, that I just don't know Jeff and he isn't doing as well as I'd hoped he was. I think I'm scared of Jeff. He was

*always someone I felt I knew so to see him change
so completely has me afraid.*

I kept Jeff home from IUP for three weeks and during that time he saw his neuropsychologist several times. We had a meeting and all decided he could go back to finish his spring classes provided he never saw or had any connection with that woman, and he said he absolutely wanted nothing to do with her again.

To my relief Jeff kept his word and did not get into any more trouble when he went back, and he passed his classes for the second semester. But he did not maintain the required B average for financial aid from DORS, so at the end of the semester Ed and I picked him up and told him he would not be returning the next year. Without the DORS financial support I could not afford it, and I now knew he needed to stay home and go to school at one of the colleges in the DC and Maryland area. I needed to keep him close by so I could know more about what he was involved with and help him when he needed me.

I felt so guilty for sending Jeff away to college before he was ready, and Ed did his best to make me feel better.

"You know, there were several positive outcomes of Jeff's year away at college," he said in his typical optimistic, reassuring manner. "One, he got to find out he could do college classes and two, he got to explore having independence and learn what college life was all about."

I had to agree with that. And I knew, or at least hoped, he learned valuable lessons about himself and how his choice of women to date might be a problem.

There was another positive outcome of the year. For the first time since Jeff's accident, without the constant distraction of Jeff and his needs, Travis and I were able to talk about his future. I wanted him to take his education more seriously, like he did when he was younger. I saw so much potential in Travis and felt he was losing sight of it.

Travis and I argued a lot about him going away to college the following year. He was going to graduate from high school soon but he assumed he had blown his chances of getting into a good university. There was some truth to it because his GPA the last two years of high school had fallen a long way. He went from being the Honor Roll student to his school counselor's worst nightmare.

"I'm not applying!" he said one day after Jeff had gone back to IUP for the spring semester and I was busy pushing Travis to fill out college applications. "No one will accept me and it's a waste of time."

I knew it was his pride talking and I was not going to give up on him.

"Travis, you need to at least try! What are you going to do if you don't go to college?" I asked him. "You need college to get a good job that you can support yourself with."

His face turned red and he clenched his fists. "I'll keep working at gas stations and work my way up," he told me. "I can be a manager."

"No! You are not going to do that!" I yelled at him, and then had to leave the room because he looked like he was so enraged with me that he might hit me. I knew he never would, but he had been lifting weights and was able to bench press two hundred fifty pounds and in his anger looked a little like the Incredible Hulk.

After we both calmed down, Travis gave in, and we sat at the kitchen table while I filled out the application forms and shoved them in front of him to sign. No matter what the outcome I just didn't want him to give up on himself. I felt that he was not entirely at fault because he was neglected during all of the drama around Jeff's brain injury and the chaos Steve and I dragged the kids through, and I wanted him to know I was still his mother and believed in him.

Jeff's year away at IUP also gave me the time to refocus on my own goals. I spent time doing literature reviews to develop my dissertation proposal even though, much like Travis and his college applications, I wasn't sure I could actually do it. After so much emotional turmoil in my life, I felt unable to do anything intellectual anymore. But one thing I knew: I could not let my ghosts from the past stop me from pursuing my dreams. When I began my psychoanalysis with Dr. Stone I told him my goal was to have a louder voice in my head that would override my father's bullying words, a voice that was encouraging and supportive, and I needed to pay attention to that new voice now.

I was so excited when I got my research proposal approved by my dissertation committee and planned to do a study of the priorities in special education for students with brain injuries. I hoped that the topic, besides giving me a way to finish my degree, would create a professional niche for me when I had the energy to return to work full time. At least it would be a step in that direction.

On May 25, 1991, not long after Jeff was home from IUP, I met with the Executive Director of the National Association of Directors of Special Education (NASDSE), Dr. William Schipper whom everyone called Skip. I had done an internship in his office for my doctoral program, and I was excited to tell Skip my research ideas. I also wanted to use the NASDSE membership, the State Directors of Special Education, for my survey. He said it was a wonderful topic and that NASDSE would help me, and he told me what I already knew, which was that I needed to talk with Dr. George Zitnay, the new President and CEO of the National Head Injury Foundation (NHIF).

"I want to talk to him but I've tried and he isn't returning my calls," I said.

Skip smiled and picked up the phone. He got through right away.

"George, Bill Schipper," he said winking at me. "There's a young lady in my office you need to meet."

That's how things are done in DC. The next day I was in Dr. George Zitnay's office and he was as full of ideas for me as if we were old friends. One of his ideas, which he said would help me with my dissertation, was that I should write a grant proposal with him so that I could work at the NHIF to help develop a national education and training program for educators about TBI. I loved that idea and didn't even try to contain my enthusiasm as I explained all of my thoughts about why this was needed and gave him examples from my personal story with Jeff.

The timing, George said, was perfect! He explained the history of the NHIF, which began in 1980 at the home of Dr. Martin Spivak and his wife Marilyn Price Spivak, who was their first Executive Director. George said that the NHIF had recently hired him away from his previous job as Director of the Kennedy Institute, to bring the NHIF to DC so they could become involved at a different level politically. He knew not only the Kennedy family but a lot of other well-connected and influential people in DC, and he said he wanted to build up the political future of brain injury research and advocacy.

I left the NHIF office that day high on adrenaline and ready to go to work, convinced that I could now create the perfect job I needed and begin my future career. At Gallaudet, as a doctoral student, one of my jobs was to help faculty write and submit grant proposals and I had discovered that I had abilities to do grant development and writing. I could do this!

George said he thought we should try to get discretionary money from the U. S. Department of Education (DOE), Office of Special Education and Rehabilitative Services (OSERS) and he would set up a meeting for us because he knew Dr. Robert Davilla, who was the Assistant Secretary of Education for OSERS. He explained that discretionary funds are those left over at the end of the fiscal year to be used at the discretion of the administrators of the agency, and that would be a quicker and simpler process than waiting for a Request for Proposals (RFP) to come out in the fall before submitting a grant application. I went home and worked all that weekend on a proposal, feeling more happy and hopeful than I had in a long time. I was so excited I could barely sleep.

We met with Dr. Davilla, on June 12. When we sat down to talk I was introduced by George through Dr. Davilla's sign language interpreter and I used my conversational sign language to remind him that we had met before.

"I thought you looked familiar," he said. I could see that he was intrigued.

"I am a doctoral student at Gallaudet and did an internship in your office one semester," I explained. Before coming to OSERS, Dr. Davilla was Dean of the Model Secondary School for the Deaf at Gallaudet.

I asked if he would prefer that I sign for myself, rather than talk through his interpreter, and when he said yes I was thrilled. We had a wonderful discussion that day about the need to prepare educational professionals to work with students with traumatic brain injuries and about Gallaudet, and I left feeling this was going to work out. I was on a high; this would lead to me having that exciting new job and help me be able to finish my Ph.D.. This was it! This was the solution I had been looking for!

Two weeks went by and we did not hear anything from OSERS, but George said to be patient and offered to hire Jeff as a receptionist for the NHIF to manage their switchboard and greet people. He thought it was a good idea to have a TBI survivor out front like that, greeting the public, and I was relieved to have Jeff employed and involved in something besides looking for women. The office was near Dupont Circle and Jeff was so proud of his new position, taking the metro downtown every day to work. The small salary covered his expenses and provided spending money for him so that he did not need to come to me for cash to support his social life. And we both met people like members of the Kennedy family, James Brady, and others who I had only seen and heard about on the news.

As Jeff began to work at the NHIF, the very place where I wanted to work, I waited to hear about my glorious new job and spent the month of June painting the house and making repairs because I needed to sell it. I had no idea where we were moving to, but we were moving. I had no choice because Steve was now fully lodged in a power play with me and continued to not pay the mortgage, saying he did not have the money even though he had somehow managed to pay for things for his girlfriend and her children.

I still had serious financial problems to deal with though and Ed was once again angry at me and worrying about his involvement with someone who he said had no ambition. No ambition? Me?

"Get a job," he told me at dinner. "Just get a job!"

I was furious and told him he obviously did not know me. I was not the person he thought I was. But I knew that the truth was that, financially speaking, my life was a mess and he was right to be concerned. I only had $195 to my name and was about to lose the house. I kept calling my lawyer, who ignored me, and I began to wonder if I would ever have the divorce agreement worked out or the money I needed to live on that the courts had awarded me. I felt I deserved the time I needed to finish my degree before getting a job, and Steve apparently thought he could force me to go back to work so he could get out of making payments.

Again I was stuck. No job, no dissertation, no final agreement or court date for my divorce, and soon no house to live in, and I couldn't pay a new attorney to help me. I felt like the walls were closing in me again and there was nothing I could do about it.

I cried a lot that summer obsessing over money, the future, whether or not I would ever have stability again, and wondering if my relationship with Ed was going to last. All I knew for certain was that I had to do whatever it took to take care of myself and my kids. There was no one else. I had to put the house up for sale and hope that it sold before the bank took it away. There was some equity in the house that would be mine if I planned it right.

We lived in a desirable neighborhood and our house was once a new, modern, beautiful family home. But now it looked like dysfunctional and depressed people lived there, which was the sad truth. The front porch pillars were broken; paint in all the rooms was chipped; we had holes in the living room walls where teenagers had smashed into them during those days no one was at home; and the carpet still smelled of dog pee two years after Christy was gone. Months of dirty dishes piling up, and no one home to clean, had taken its toll; roaches had begun moving in as if they were the new home owners. I did not have the money to hire an exterminator or have the carpets professionally cleaned so I had to do it myself with cans of bug spray and carpet shampoo. It was not very effective.

I was afraid that the house was such a disaster it would never sell, but I was equally terrified that it would sell because I had no idea how I would find a new place with no income. I wasn't even sure a real estate agent could help but I had to sell it or lose it. I found a sympathetic woman named Michelle who said she would list it for me and offered suggestions for fixing the house up with almost no money. I listed the house for sale, and people came to see it, but I got no offers as the hot, miserable, muggy summer dragged on and came to an end.

The good news was that Travis was accepted at one of the three universities he applied to, which surprised him and motivated him to go to college even though he did not want to go to the college that had accepted him. We decided he would live at home and get an associate's degree from the nearby community college. Then he could transfer to the University of Maryland without his high school transcripts being a factor.

Somehow Ed and I survived the summer, and Jeff and Travis both went back to school at the community college in September. I tried to not let the kids know how afraid I was that we might lose the house and relied on Ed and my psychiatrist to listen to my fears. Most of the time Ed was supportive but there were times he went back to telling me I should find a job and that would solve the problem.

On September 2, in the middle of the night, I could not sleep and was hysterical crying in that out of control, unable to stop way I had when Jeff was first hurt. I told Ed the world was coming to an end because I could not pay for anything we needed, and we were going to be evicted from our home and living in a shelter at this rate.

"What can I do?" I cried.

Half asleep, his eyes still closed, he yawned and said, "Put it all in a God Box."

"What the hell is that?" I yelled at him. "Is that another one of your stupid twelve step things?" I was so mad at him; how could he be so insensitive? "God isn't going to help me with this!"

"Just try it because, you know, your way isn't working." He yawned.

"Okay, well how? I don't believe in God and don't know how to do that!" I was working myself up into a frenzy, and I knew I was taking out my frustrations on the very person who really loved me and was trying to help me. I told myself I needed to calm down but I couldn't.

"I don't know," he said. "Maybe you can picture a box, maybe a golden one, and put all your problems in there. Turn it all over and then try to go back to sleep."

He reached for my hand and as he held on I pictured a golden box in the air above me and all of my problems, one by one, going in there. I was desperate so I did what he suggested even though I thought it was all a bunch of hooey. And I did go back to sleep.

To my surprise, more people began coming to see the house the next day and on September 14, twelve days after the God Box experiment, I got an offer to buy the house. The offer was from an Army Chaplain no less, and Ed just smiled smugly and said, "See? It works. "

Later that same day I got an even better offer for the full asking price of the house, and I signed a contract. This was enough to make me think there really was something to this idea of turning problems over to God or a Higher Power.

Michelle had to call Steve to get his signature on the contract because the house was still joint property, and I resented that he would benefit from the sale since it I felt it was his fault we had to sell it in the first place. Also I was the one who had worked to get it ready, spending my days and evenings spackling holes in the walls, painting, and fixing broken things that he was not there to help with.

According to state divorce laws I knew we should be able to stay in our home for two years while I got on my feet, but that was not a realistic option now. What made it bearable to me was that I knew Steve owed me a lot of back child support and other money, and when I calculated the amounts I saw with the glee of divorce revenge that he would not get money from the house sale anyway.

Steve called me, wanting to talk, and we met at a Subway restaurant where we had a long, comfortable conversation for the first time in several years. We agreed that this divorce did not need to be so adversarial and decided to fire our attorneys and work together on an amicable rewritten settlement agreement. He said he felt guilty for all he'd done and agreed to pay me all of the money he now owed me. In exchange, I let him out of any future support payments even though Jeff's disability meant Steve could be required to pay child support to me for the rest of Jeff's life. I did not want any financial ties to Steve ever again.

"I still love you, but I am not in love with you and don't want to be married to you," I said with a smile. "I think we are doing the right thing getting a divorce."

He reached for my hand across the table and smiled back at me. "I agree and I love you too." Of course he did. He wanted money. He tried to convince me to give him some of the proceeds from the sale of the house to help "a friend" he owed money to, and I said no.

When I left the Subway I knew that eventually I would forgive him, but I also knew I would never trust him again. And knowing that felt real, and good, and safe. I knew I could take care of myself now which was something Steve and my parents had led me to believe I couldn't do.

At that point our divorce felt like it meant more than just doing the right thing; it let me smash walls and open doors to the rest of my life. But I also knew I would always miss the young, idealistic love relationship I thought we had at one time. It wasn't real, but I would miss it.

Steve and I were divorced on October 3, 1991 in a simple, uncontested hearing at the Rockville Courthouse with no lawyers and only my friend Judy as a witness to verify that we had been separated the required length of time.

"Do you believe this couple has differences that are irreconcilable?" the judge asked her.

She looked at me and smiled. "Yes, absolutely," she said. And that was all it took. Our marriage of twenty-two years was over. I decided to go back to my maiden name of Ruoff and start my new future, which I hoped would include me with my Ph.D., a healthy Jeff, a more focused Travis, and Ed.

In November I found a beautiful townhouse not far from where we had been living, and the landlord agreed to rent it to me because I showed her my signed final divorce agreement saying I would get all of the back money Steve owed me from the proceeds of the sale of our house. By Christmas of 1991 I was exhausted but happy because I was finally divorced, living in a new place of my own with my two almost grown sons, and we even had a small Christmas tree.

I felt like I was on the way to getting that new life I had wanted for so long. Ed was relieved that I actually was divorced now and not just talking about it because, it turned out, he felt that it was morally wrong to be dating someone who was still married. I had no idea he felt that way and laughed at him for it. "Everyone dates when they are separated," I told him.

Ed began spending time during the week as well as weekends at my new house and we grew closer if that was even possible. He encouraged me to work a little every day on my dissertation, and I set up a small table with a computer at the end of the kitchen. When I wasn't reading my endless supply of self-help books, or going to therapy, I spent my time at that computer determined to continue to make progress with my research.

In terms of finding a job I still felt I was stuck, though. It was becoming clear to me that the NHIF project was not going to work; I was disappointed but tried to stay positive and hopeful. George said that he still thought we could work together to build a training program that I could oversee.

But then he called me one day to give me the bad news.

"Janis, I'm sorry but we are not going to do the training program," he said. "The George Washington University has submitted a grant proposal to start a new graduate training program in TBI and Special Education and our Pediatric Task Force is supporting it."

I was stunned and disappointed beyond words. I couldn't talk so I just listened as he went on with his other ideas for me.

"You could still help us with some of the things we are working on, and you should give GW a call," he said. "Maybe you could work with them."

I thanked him and hung up in tears, feeling the sense of defeat and hopelessness creeping into my body once again. Why should I call people at GW when I was mad at them for stealing my project? And besides, I was pretty sure that no one at a major university like that would want to have me involved when I hadn't finished my Ph.D. yet.

I ignored George's suggestion and went back into my familiar dark hole of grief and abandonment. Another door had closed in my face and I saw no other doors opening so what next? I turned to Ed for help.

"You need a job, and you need to finish your dissertation," he said.

It was true. The time had come for me to get out of the passive position of expecting someone else to help me with my professional goals. I had broken through my walls and now I needed to figure out how to get to that greener pasture I'd been in search of for so long. I had to do the looking, the sniffing out of greener grass, and make my own decisions.

I began applying for jobs that I saw advertised in the Washington Post but nothing came of it so while I was waiting I spent time every day on my dissertation. I started with thirty minutes and worked up to two hours a day, and before long I was making progress.

I remember occasional times when I was taking a public bus to the community college I went to, before and after IUP, and I would often get off at the wrong stop and have to walk the rest of the way, maybe a mile or so, to school. Once I even got off the bus at a shopping center, became confused as to why I was there and applied for a job at one of the retail stores. I have a hard time remembering how I felt about things during that time of my life (it was about two decades ago) but I do know I felt a great deal of frustration, anxiety, and embarrassment.

—Jeff Bouck, TBI Survivor

Chapter 7

A New Family Dance

I ONCE DID A PRESENTATION on the learning process after a TBI and described it as a dance with one step forward and two back, which I envision as a kind of a hip-hop waltz. The whole family begins to dance that way after someone has a brain injury. In 1989 I didn't fully understand that our family's dance had just begun and that we had a lifetime of waltzing crazily through time ahead of us. We were all learning a new dance but there was no instructor. And it seemed at times like Jeff was in the lead with no idea what the steps were or even what dance he was doing. He was like some of the guys I met at singles dances who had too much to drink and just walked around the dance floor, oblivious to the music, expecting me to follow them.

I was getting used to this life though, and for the most part I was content as I worked on my dissertation part of each day, applied for more jobs, and spent the rest of the time reading a lot of self-help books, going to therapy appointments, and enjoying my time with Ed when I could.

My new townhouse was within walking distance of a metro stop and just a few miles from the community college, so Jeff and Travis left in the mornings to go to school or work and returned in the evenings. Ed spent the weekends with us and he and I talked every night on the phone during the week. Life had a pleasant hum to it now.

Jeff seemed to like his job at the NHIF. He liked taking the metro there every day and being at the front desk when important people came to see Dr. Zitnay. He also liked answering the phones and talking to people, and unfortunately he liked it a little too much. When a young lady named Lilly began calling the NHIF looking for information about TBI, because she was a TBI survivor, Jeff was at the switchboard and took her calls. And then he began accepting her collect phone calls every day after that and developing a relationship with her.

About two weeks after he told us about Lilly, Jeff came home from work and announced that he and his buddy, a friend from high school who also had a TBI, were going to drive to Pittsburgh to meet her. I argued with him but he insisted this was important and took off in a snowstorm before I had time to stop him. Ed and I laughed but at the same time I thought: oh, no here we go again! I had flashbacks to the relationship he had at IUP that caused him so much trouble, but for Jeff it seemed to be totally unrelated to Lilly and his new romance.

Jeff made it home the next day, and after that trip Lilly became a part of our life. She began to spontaneously take the bus from Pittsburgh to visit us for a few days at a time, and she continued to call Jeff at the NHIF constantly when she was back home. We liked Lilly, and she was not at all like his IUP con artist, but I knew Jeff needed to focus on his job and taking Lilly's calls at work was a big distraction.

It was also a problem in other ways as I soon found out. George called me one day to say that he was concerned about Jeff accepting the collect calls from this girl because it was running up a large phone bill, and he asked that I come to the NHIF to meet with him and Jeff's supervisor.

"We don't know what to do," Jeff's supervisor told me when we had our meeting. "We are going to have to take money from his paycheck to pay for these calls."

"Go ahead," I told them. "And I'll talk to him about it again. But he does have memory problems you know. Couldn't you just change his responsibilities so he's not answering the phones?"

He said no, they could not do that; apparently they just wanted someone to do what Jeff was assigned to do and didn't want to make changes for him. I was shocked that people on staff of the leading organization for advocacy and information about brain injury could not figure out what to do to supervise someone like Jeff who had the impaired judgment and memory problems of a young TBI survivor. And I resented being pulled into it.

In March, 1992 Ed, Jeff, Lilly and I took the metro into DC to attend the first ever NHIF rally for TBI on Capitol Hill, which I thought was an event we would enjoy. We were all excited about taking part in what we believed was an historical event for TBI. But the minute I got there an NHIF staff member pounced on me, complaining about Jeff, and then Jeff and Lilly did not want to participate in the rally so we left early.

Not long after the Capitol Hill rally, Jeff was fired. It was my first lesson on how hard it is for a person with a brain injury to receive job supports that work out for everyone. I sympathized with the NHIF's dilemma. Jeff's actions were costing them money, and they operated on a bare bones budget anyway, but I thought there should have been something they could do to keep Jeff on. As it turned out Jeff didn't care as much as I did, and I realized he moved on to new things better than I did in a lot of ways. His focus now was on dating Lilly, not on keeping a job I thought he should want.

Maybe, I thought, my problem was that I focused too much on managing Jeff's life when I really need to better manage mine? I was getting new insight all the time into how much I did that and I was just glad to still have my regular therapy appointments with Dr. Stone.

"I don't know what kind of work I want to do," I told him. "I had a plan but it's not looking like that's working out. So now what?" The one thing I knew for sure was that I had to find a job, any job, sooner rather than later.

I was beginning to understand that any future work I did in the field of brain injury was going to be hard for me because of my personal involvement and my emotional reactions. While I wanted to be objective and understand that dealing with Jeff was not easy, the truth was that I wanted to protect him from being hurt in any way after all he'd been through. Would my life ever settle down? I was still tired and run down from the exhausting year before, and beginning to question if I would ever find a job, finish my dissertation, and if Jeff would ever make it to being an independent adult.

It felt like I was doing pointless work and Ed was wonderful at propping me up and telling me to take things one day at a time. I was raised on a steady diet of ruminating about the past and worrying about the future. I don't think my parents ever talked about the here and now except to discuss housework or family activities. It was like Ed was speaking a foreign language to me but I was beginning to understand words and phrases now and then.

Even though I was disappointed with the way things had worked out for Jeff, I wanted to maintain my relationship with George and the NHIF so I agreed to help them when I could, on a volunteer basis, and one day George called to ask for my help with one of their projects.

"We are working with Senator Edward Kennedy on a new piece of legislation," he said. "It's called the Traumatic Brain Injury Act and I'd like for you to read drafts and send me your ideas and comments."

He explained the complicated process of getting a bill passed and I was eager to help because it sounded like legislation that could someday be helpful to people like our family. But I also knew I needed to stay focused on finishing my Ph.D. and job search. About a month later I was offered a position as director of speech therapy programs for a large nursing and rehabilitation center in Virginia. I was afraid of going back to work in the field of speech-language therapy but it was a job with a steady income that would pay the bills and would give me that stability I knew I needed.

I talked to Dr. Stone about it and he asked what I was worried about.

"I just don't know if I can do it," I said in tears. "It was becoming emotionally draining for me to be with people so needy all of the time even before Jeff's TBI and now..."

I stopped because I wasn't even sure exactly what I was afraid of. Losing myself in the process of trying to solve other people's problems? Giving up the time to work on my dissertation? Never being able to say no when someone needed my help? It was all of that and more.

"But you have boundaries now that you didn't have then," he reminded me.

True, I did. And I did love helping people; it was as easy for me as planning vacations was for Ed. Helping just always came naturally to me even as a young child. So I accepted the job and quickly I came to love what I was doing.

Jeff didn't pay much attention to my new job but Travis did, and when I saw him looking so relieved that I was employed again I realized how hard this must have been for him during the years of having to take on part-time jobs while going to school.

Travis was doing well in college and seemed to have a new sense of purpose. He was excited about becoming an engineer and determined to make it work so that he could go to the University of Maryland. Then one day he came home and told me he had met a girl named Becky and he really liked her.

"Mom, she is the nicest girl I have ever known," he said and then he chuckled. "She's probably too nice for me."

A few months later Jeff broke up with Lilly and began dating a girl named Mimi who turned out to be a friend of Becky's. We became like a blended family and Ed and I enjoyed spending time with all of the kids. I loved the feeling of family life again, and I wanted more. I was beginning to think I could get married again, and maybe to Ed.

In July, 1992, on a hot and muggy east coast summer night, Ed and I were on the phone to say goodnight as we always did before going to sleep.

"It's so hot here," he said. "I can't sleep." He owned a small, older house with no central air conditioning.

"That's too bad. It's nice here," I said, enjoying teasing him. "But of course I have air conditioning." I paused. "Why don't you come over?"

"Why don't I just come over and stay?" he said.

And that's how we began living together. Ed is a cautious person and moved in slowly, one change of clothes at a time, until a few months later we signed a joint lease on the townhouse with both of our names on it. That next Christmas he presented me with an engagement ring and we celebrated by taking Jeff and Travis on a three-day trip to the Bahamas.

In January 1993 we returned from a wonderful engagement trip to phone messages from my bother saying, "Dad's had a stroke, call me." Then there was one last call left on the night we returned saying just "call me."

When I called my brother in Texas he told me that our father had been pronounced brain dead from a severe brain stem stroke and they had decided to take him off life support. He was gone and the funeral would be the next morning.

"What? You planned the funeral without me?" I said. My head was reeling from the shock of my father's death and the sense of betrayal upon learning that no one considered me an important part of family decisions anymore. It was the price of speaking up for myself, and I was not prepared.

To my amazement, my brother told me I should not come to the funeral, that it was not appropriate "under the circumstances," and that my mother did not want me there. "It's for her, after all," he said. Knowing I didn't matter, as always, sent me into a sea of guilt and remorse. I thought maybe I should not have pushed back against the abuse my father heaped on me. Maybe I should have just smiled and said nothing to keep the peace like I did as a child.

I plunged into old familiar childhood shame, panic attacks, and nightmares that I had lived with my whole life. My father was gone and despite our arguments I loved him and I knew he would have wanted us all there at his bedside and at his funeral. I wanted to be there, I needed to be. But it was too late.

There was nothing I could do about the funeral; I was not wanted and so I would not go. It took weeks of crying and beating up on myself, and a few intense therapy sessions, but I eventually saw that being left out of my own father's funeral was a kind of validation for me. I had always doubted my perceptions but now it was clear to me that I did not imagine the degrading way my parents and brother discounted me all my life. Who tells someone they aren't welcome at her own father's funeral? I couldn't change the past or even how they treated me now, but I could change how I reacted. I could react by taking care of myself and my kids and our need to say goodbye to someone we all loved.

I could hold my own funeral for my Dad. I organized a small memorial service at my townhouse and I put out all the pictures I had of my father with me, the kids, and other family members. I invited my friends, and I presented a eulogy that I wrote, and I gave Jeff and Travis time to say a few words about their grandfather. They needed to have the chance to grieve and share their memories because he may not have been the best father to me but he was a wonderful grandfather. That memorial service was a turning point for me because I felt empowered; I had a voice now and I did not have to allow people to mistreat me or push me aside anymore.

Once again I was so grateful to have Ed with me because our relationship was completely grounded in reality, unlike most of the relationships I had known before. I got through that dark period of time committed even more than ever to doing all of the things I needed to do to keep that promise to God, the vow I made when I was recovering from surgery in 1989 and afraid I might die.

That spring new professional opportunities came my way and I was excited to be moving in the direction I wanted, becoming more involved with the field of brain injury. In addition to my job in the nursing and rehabilitation center, I was asked to be on a board for a TBI brain injury case management program in northern Virginia. And through connections I made with that organization I was given an opportunity to work privately as a cognitive therapist with a young lady who was Deaf and had a brain injury.

Being so active again, I felt I was returning to my old self and moments of real happiness were beginning to pop up for me like small splashes of bright red and orange across a canvas that had only shown images of gray and black clouds before.

The lease on the townhouse was ending and Ed and I began talking about where we wanted to live after we were married. We decided we needed a place of our own where we could start our new life as a married couple. We began house hunting, an activity I always enjoy, but we didn't find anything. I wanted a place big enough that Jeff and Travis could continue living with us for a few more years, to give them the stable family life I felt they had been deprived of, and we both wanted to be close enough to the metro and the DC Beltway that our commuting to work would be reasonable. And we agreed we wanted a new house so we didn't have to spend too much time fixing it up.

"I think we should have a house built, one that we pick out together and design to be ours," I said. Ed agreed and we selected a neighborhood in Silver Spring not far from where he had lived all of his life.

After the foundation for our new home was laid we stood in the front yard staring at it in awe and talking about our appreciation for all that we had in our lives. Ed was a lonely bachelor when I met him and I had so many problems in my life that the idea of a second marriage seemed remote and something I might never want even if the opportunity presented itself. How did this happen? We were both in tears remembering our beginnings and how far we'd come together.

We moved into our new house with Jeff and Travis in July, 1994 and Ed and I were married on September 17. The weeks surrounding our wedding were almost surreal as we spent time getting ready, enjoying the company of old friends and the community we had created together, and putting our futures together in a wedding ceremony that we designed ourselves and made our own. A large man from Trinidad, who worked with Ed, sang "One in a Million You" and we had a reception at a nearby rhythm and blues club where I danced the entire time.

When we returned from our honeymoon cruise in the Caribbean I began the vigil of finishing a dissertation; staying up late every night to write and rewrite sections, binging on junk food as I always did when stressed, and gaining weight but deliriously happy to be doing all of the things I had wanted to do and thought I couldn't in 1989.

In the spring of 1995 I presented my dissertation research to my faculty committee and university administrators, with Ed and Judy attending to give me support. That morning, before we left for Gallaudet, I was so nervous I told Ed I just couldn't do it. I felt sick thinking of all the years of work and I had so much anxiety I thought I would throw up. All those years and all of the pain and suffering, and now it seemed my whole life hinged on my performance that day.

"You can do it," Ed said. "You are meant to be Dr. Ruoff." I wondered how did I get so lucky to find someone like him? I didn't know why, but it was clear that he believed in me more than I did.

The chair of my department, Dr. Bill Marshall, made a speech at the end of my dissertation defense to congratulate me.

"Some of you may not know this," he said, signing as he spoke in his loud and commanding voice, "but Dr. Ruoff would have been dead in the water in two more hours!"

It turned out that I finished my Ph.D. just two hours before my statute of limitations would have run out. If I had known that I probably would have gone into a fetal position and never made it to my dissertation defense or I would have become frozen when asked questions. You just never know what you can do until you try. All the years my father laughed at me and called me an idiot, stupid, or shithead were beginning to be erased when I got my Ph.D.. I think a lot of people go for advanced degrees as ghost-busters; I know I did. It was like Ed with his CP and sports. He was proving to himself he could do something physical, much like I needed to prove to myself that I was more than just a cute girl child who was silly and overly emotional.

That night as I lay in bed I imagined talking to the ghost of my father who so often called me names and made fun of me just for being a girl. In my vision I showed him my degree and said, "That's Doctor Shithead to you!" I think he would have laughed and offered me a drink to that.

I went through a "getting real with my parents" phase in my twenties and decided I wanted to distance from my mother and work on my relationship with my dad, who I had never been close to. I asked him why he never said he loved me my entire life, and why he was so mean and critical toward me. He said he wasn't good with emotions and had assumed I knew he loved me, and that the reason he insulted me was to make me a better person. He said that was how the coaches he had admired when he was a high school athlete had pushed him. He also said he didn't want me to be conceited. Conceited? I had such low self-esteem I did not see how he could have been worried about that!

After those conversations, I knew that in his own misguided way he treated me like he did to encourage me; it was his warped way of showing love. I missed fighting with my father. He was a harsh coach, and I needed more sensitivity, but I think he secretly wanted me to be successful and independent. He just did not know how to encourage that for me as a woman because both he and my mother were products of an era that believed women should be subservient to men and taken care of by men.

The interesting thing about finishing a Ph.D. is that the next day you are still you, and I was back to work in a nursing home helping people with their communication and swallowing problems, pushing wheelchairs around and waiting while someone took twenty minutes to go to the bathroom in the middle of our therapy session. It was a good reminder to stay humble.

I'm a person who seems to love to create new complications for myself. The challenge of completing my dissertation was over, my family life seemed relatively calm for the moment, and my work was becoming routine. So I began thinking about new goals. I even considered applying to law school thinking I might become a disability rights lawyer.

A few weeks after I defended my dissertation, I summoned up my courage and called Theresa Krankowski, who ran the grant-funded program in TBI and special education at George Washington University.

"Hi, you don't know me but my name is Janis Ruoff and I'm interested in teaching about TBI," I began. She didn't hang up on me so I continued.

"My son had a TBI a few years ago and I did my dissertation on the current status of special education and TBI, and I would love to meet with you and hear about the program at GW."

"Thank you for calling!" she said, much to my surprise. "You are an answer to my prayers!"

I was not sure what I expected when I called Theresa but I was relieved and touched that she was so happy to hear from me. I laughed.

"How am I an answer to your prayers?" I asked.

"I have all of this work to do with coordinating the grant and I'm a doctoral student too, and I'm just overwhelmed. I need help and I think you could be just what I need. When can you come over here?"

The next day I took off from work and went to her office in the basement of the infamous Watergate Hotel in DC. We had a wonderful conversation about teaching and what the field of TBI needed and all of the things I was so excited about. Theresa then set up another meeting for me to join her with her faculty advisor, Dr. Carol Kochhar, and after they checked my background I was hired to teach the next semester as an adjunct professor. I was so excited as I prepared to teach my first class at a major university.

But then it all fell apart because that spring there were not enough students signed up for my first class, and it was cancelled. It was just my introduction to the realities of university teaching, but at the time I took it personally. I assumed I wasn't wanted.

"Don't worry, we do want you to teach in the fall," Theresa assured me, but I didn't believe it. I was reminded of the NHIF experience, and disappointing times when I was a child and I got excited about something I might get to do that never materialized. I became depressed again, wondering why people put opportunities in front of me only to snatch them away. I wanted so much now to be let into this world of universities, something I had dreamed of many years before but put out of my mind as unreachable. Were walls always going to pop up in my life just when I thought I was free to go in the direction I wanted to?

"How do I get in?" I asked Dave Martin when we met for dinner one evening. I trusted Dave's advice. He was one of the smartest and most successful people I knew and I still thought of him as my mentor.

He thought for a minute. "Well, some universities are easier than others to become involved with. But you just hang around and do whatever they need. Just be involved however you can and do stuff."

Just do stuff? Okay, I could do that! I continued to meet with Theresa and Carol and offered to help supervise a few projects students were working on, and I tried to give Theresa the emotional support she needed to manage all of her responsibilities and coursework. I was doing what Dave had advised me to do: just hang around and do stuff, and I was getting to know these people and helping them to be more comfortable with me because, after all, I was an outsider. I also continued to stay in touch with Dr. Zitnay and help the NHIF in whatever way I could.

I was invited to attend the NHIF's annual conference in June, 1995 and was there for their announcement that they were changing their name to the Brain Injury Association of America, and I got to meet more of the people who were leaders in the growing field of brain injury advocacy. I submitted a proposal to present my research at a national conference and waited.

My presentation proposal was accepted and in December of that year I presented my dissertation at a brain injury conference in San Diego, California where I met the researchers I had quoted in my literature review and who I so admired for their pioneering work in traumatic brain injury. I was like a kid in a candy store getting to be involved in what I had longed for since Jeff's accident, but had felt was above me. Even though Jeff was still struggling with his life and independence maybe I now had a voice in the professional world of TBI that I hoped I could use it to make a difference for him and others like him.

As I stood up to begin my presentation I was told that they were running out of time because the group before me had gone over their time. I only had ten minutes. That threw me for a loop because I had worked on this study for years and had so much I wanted to say. I introduced myself and my topic and told them I was also the mother of a young TBI survivor. The room was so quiet it was unnerving.

"At our house the family joke is that Jeff had his TBI just to give me my dissertation topic because I didn't know what to do it on."

No one laughed. I saw looks of pity on their faces, and that was not what I wanted.

"It's okay, you can laugh. We do," I said. There were a few smiles then and I did the fastest overview I could, covering just the main points of my research and asking for questions. Someone in the audience who I recognized as a leader in the field, Dr. Ron Savage, who I had quoted the most in my dissertation literature review, raised his hand. I gulped. I knew who he was and imagined he was going to say my study was terrible and insult me like my father might have. But he wasn't my father.

"That was the best dissertation presentation I ever heard!" he said with a big smile meaning, I was sure, that it was short and to the point. Wow; these people didn't think my ideas were stupid! I felt that I was getting the respect I had craved my whole life. I was on cloud nine.

In the fall of 1996 I began teaching classes at GW and supervising students who were doing their internships. Gradually I became known in the brain injury community as a faculty member for the Master's degree in special education and TBI, the very program that George Zitnay had told me about in 1991. After years of resenting that program and the faculty for what I had perceived as taking away my dream, I was now a part of it. It's a funny thing about resentments. I was learning that for me resentment was often rooted in jealousy because I was just not allowing myself to pursue what I wanted in life. When I did, when I broke through my walls of pride and fear, those resentments melted away with the bricks and mortar left behind.

Classes were taught in the evenings at GW so I could still work in nursing homes and schools during the day. After a few months I quit my full time job so that I could have a flexible schedule and be available to help more at GW, and I negotiated a contract with the corporate office of the nursing homes to be a PRN, or as-needed, speech pathologist. I also arranged a contract with the local school district to help with their speech therapy needs in two middle schools that were understaffed. It was all working out and I couldn't believe it at times. I had the husband I wanted, the career I wanted, and my health was returning to normal.

I was happy with so much of my life, but so worried about Jeff that it was hard for me to teach about brain injury knowing that my own son needed help but people, including me, didn't know how to help him.

Sometimes I would cry all the way home after a class that touched on the painful reality of life for someone after a TBI. Especially when I talked about Jeff's problems as an example, or when we had guest speakers who were struggling with similar difficulties. I felt like I was immersed full time, around the clock, in the subject of TBI. I longed for a break. There were times I thought maybe it was a mistake to wrap my professional work around the same thing causing me so much trouble at home, and maybe I should have switched paths. But whenever I thought about, or tried, to pull back on my work with brain injury something kept me stuck. I felt like a fly caught in a spider web. The more I saw Jeff experiencing so many ups and downs in his life, the more passionate I was about changing the world through educating others about TBI and the pervasive, sometimes subtle effects of an injury to the brain on the person and everyone around him.

Jeff seemed to be falling farther and farther down a rabbit hole that left him confused and unable to move toward any goals he had. At times he didn't even remember he had goals, and he was happy living in the moment no matter how crazy I saw it was; at other times he just seemed lost and depressed.

The obvious contrast between Jeff and Travis around education and work was growing and we all saw it at home. While Travis was doing very well at the University of Maryland and entering his chosen career field of Civil Engineering, Jeff's problems with employment kept him from moving into any kind of career that would support him and help him gain the independence that he saw his brother was achieving. I knew how much that bothered Jeff, and it was sad to watch them growing apart, but I wanted Travis to have all of the success he could without feeling any survivor's guilt.

"Jeff, you have to remember you each have your own path," I told him when he made comments that suggested he thought he was a failure compared to Travis or his old friends who also were finishing their degrees. "You will get there but just on your own time schedule."

But the question was where? Where would he get to? He was still living at home going from one job to another and one relationship to another. He kept trying to go to school but finally quit taking classes after one expensive semester at American University where he failed everything.

"You got all Fs?" I asked him incredulously when I saw his grades. "What happened?"

"I don't know," he said with that confused look he got when he couldn't remember events and make sense of what had happened to him. I made an appointment with the academic advisor he worked with, and we went together for a meeting.

"He failed because he just didn't go to classes," the counselor said. "Jeff was doing some kind of volunteer work with the English as a second language program on campus." She looked at him as if expecting an explanation, and of course he responded with a blank stare, looking embarrassed. He was like the young child who has done something wrong and who can't explain why he did it.

The Army has an expression: SOS. Same old shit. Some people say same song, second verse. It was a different version of the same story over and over; Jeff got distracted by something that made him feel good about himself and took very little effort. Jeff had volunteered to teach English to the janitorial staff and focused all of his energies on that instead of his school work. I saw that it made him feel like a big shot to walk across campus and hear the guys call out "Hola Señor Jeff!"

The worst part for me, besides the three thousand dollars I spent for nothing that semester, was that he had lied to me again. I knew nothing about his volunteer work until it was too late.

"Let's bag college for a year or so and you just get a job," I told him when Ed and I discussed things with Jeff that night. He seemed relieved and set out to find a new job instead of going to school, and he was always good at charming people and convincing them he could do things he couldn't so he got hired over and over. He just couldn't keep the jobs.

I incurred my brain injury at the age of eighteen and, like most people that age, was an expert at living in denial of my shortfalls. I would get retail jobs working as a cashier when I was unable to develop a working memory of the geography of the store. I had impulse control problems and developed a habit of beginning relationships with fellow employees that were not allowed by company policies. I would also be unable to remember my work schedules but, because I was unable to accept my memory problems, I rarely wrote down the weekly schedules and would be chronically absent and/or tardy for work. All of these problems resulted in my losing jobs just about as quickly as I could get them.

—Jeff Bouck, TBI Survivor

Chapter 8

The Plan Isn't Working

WE HAD A PLAN: The Plan for Jeff's Future. It seemed simple to me that he could find a job he liked and that would motivate him to go back to school and pursue some sort of career. We were all willing to help him, and I had a lot of connections to get him professional services and supports if he needed it. He was twenty-five now and was still a smart person despite his cognitive challenges. I could not figure out why he couldn't make this work out, or what I needed to do to help him.

While I had a feeling of gut-wrenching frustration at times, Ed and I also had a lot of good laughs over Jeff's "job of the week." The funniest was when he announced that he was hired with Maid Brigade. After a few days he came home all excited because they made him a supervisor.

"Why would they do that?" I asked. "You have never ever, maybe in your entire life, even cleaned your own room!" I laughed so hard I almost wet my pants.

"I think it's because I speak English and some Spanish and most of the maids speak Spanish," he said turning red. "And I'm a guy." Good insight, I thought. That job lasted almost two weeks.

Over the next two years he must have had a hundred different jobs, mostly part-time sales positions with no benefits. Because he was an adult, and too old for us to put him on our insurance, that meant he had no health care coverage. Theoretically the military was supposed to provide lifetime medical care for someone permanently disabled before the age of twenty-three while his parent was an active duty service member, but a technicality when I submitted the application caused Jeff to be denied.

The problem was that the Department of Defense form required that I say Jeff was financially supported more than fifty percent by the service member, Steve, and that was not true. I was the one supporting him. I refused to lie on a federal form even though Steve and someone with the Department of Defense encouraged me to do so. A few years later I filed a congressional complaint to get him reinstated with health care through the military but even Congresswoman Connie Morella's office could not get it changed.

Getting Jeff government benefits and supports as someone with a disability was a constant source of frustration in my life and I began to see similar problems with the larger population of all people disabled from a TBI. I became determined to do something about that but I wasn't sure what at the time. I was learning so much as I tried to get help for Jeff through government agencies and resources, but even though I was now on national committees and getting to know people in high places it was a problem that seemed insurmountable.

Qualifying for government benefits, I was learning, is a screwed up, complicated process with traumatic brain injury partly because many people after a TBI can function in a seemingly normal, independent manner for periods of time but cannot sustain it. The effects of a TBI are not consistent like they might be with other kinds of disabilities. TBI doesn't fit neatly into the checkboxes of government forms with categories such as deaf, blind, mentally retarded (now intellectually disabled), or physically disabled. Each person is affected differently by a TBI depending on what type of injury, what part of the brain is damaged, and other factors. Some people have cognitive challenges, some having physical disabilities, some have impairments of vision or hearing, and some have a combination of all or some of them. Added to that are also the psychological problems associated with brain injury such as PTSD and depression.

TBI is like a moving target so lawmakers and those in authority positions for government programs, and those who implement the programs; don't understand brain injury; hence my crusade to educate the world about the effects of TBI. The world did not "get it" when it came to TBI; that was what we always said when those of us involved with brain injury advocacy got together.

But my primary focus at that time was to help Jeff. He would have qualified for Social Security Disability Insurance (SSDI) and the state health care through Medicaid, based on low income, except that he kept finding employment just long enough for the government to decide he could take care of himself. He had an income, so every time he applied for SSDI, he was disqualified. It was constant chaos and I was terrified that he would have serious health problems, or another car accident, and Ed and I would go broke trying to help him.

I felt bad that Ed, who was not even Jeff's biological father, was put in the position of so much financial responsibility for Jeff. But Ed said he loved Jeff and felt like his dad so it was okay with him. Ed's commitment to Jeff made me even more grateful for him, and our relationship kept me sane and grounded through all of the craziness that my life included at that time.

As Theresa Krankowski finished her own dissertation and was ready to move on to other pursuits, I was told the brain injury program at GW would be ending soon because other faculty members had their own priorities. They had voted against submitting a new grant proposal for the program because no one wanted to work on it. I did not want to accept that decision, so I set up an appointment to talk to Carol Kochhar.

"What can I do to help?" I asked Carol. I knew she understood the need for the program, but she said there was nothing we could do until some other time.

In early May of 1997 I taught the last class on TBI at GW and left in tears. As I walked across the campus to the parking lot I talked with a few students and we all agreed that it was unfair.

"Dr. Ruoff you have to do something," one of them told me. "You can save this program!"

My savior complex was completely triggered by those words and the feeling that it was all up to me kept me up at nights. I tried to explain to the students that I did not have full tenure track faculty status at GW and I wasn't sure there was anything I could do, but I knew that I was not going to give up that easily.

I continued to badger Carol and the next year we submitted a new grant proposal to the U.S. Department of Education to start a new Master's degree program in brain injury and special education with me as the Project Director. A few months later, however, we learned that it was not funded. I was crushed and felt defeated once again.

I decided I would not give up but had to earn money in the meantime. Unlike previous years I was not confused or lost regarding my professional goals, what I considered to be my purpose now. And I did have some income-producing work. I still had my contract work with the nursing homes, which paid reasonably well, and the contract with the local school district doing speech pathology work in middle schools.

I was busy with that work, and with brain injury boards and committees that I had been asked to join, but I was set on getting back to teaching at GW. So, in keeping with Dave Martin's advice about just hanging around and doing stuff, I continued to teach other courses at GW whenever they needed me to.

I also knew that political changes were occurring related to traumatic brain injury. A new Congressional Task Force on TBI had been formed with a lot of bipartisan members of Congress signing on, and I hoped new work opportunities would come up as a result. In 1996 the TBI Act that I had helped the NHIF with in 1991 was finally passed by Congress. The appropriations for that legislation would make money available to the Health Resources Services Administration (HRSA) to fund new state programs for people with brain injuries.

In the summer of 1997 I was asked to be a grant reviewer for the first round of state grant proposals that were submitted to the HRSA for funding from the TBI Act. Wow, I was so excited to be a part of the end results of a political process I had been involved with since its infancy! I was seeing how politics and the work of our government happened, and it was about people like us, our family, to help us have a better life.

The grant review was held at a hotel in Bethesda where I spent two days reading proposals and voting to recommend whether to fund them or not. At the end of the grant review process I stood in the lobby of that hotel and talked with my friends and fellow reviewers. They were as committed to the cause as I was. We were so full of hope that the government grants would help the states who received them to improve their supports and services for people and families dealing with TBI. I couldn't wait to see what impact this would have on real people like Jeff.

As we stood in that hotel lobby talking, one of my friends asked me "Janis, why didn't Maryland submit a proposal?"

I didn't have an answer and just shook my head. I had no idea why my own state was not one of the applicants. I knew firsthand that the state needed the help. Maybe with better coordination of supports for people like Jeff he would not be floundering and unable to keep a job.

"I have to do something about this," I said, half to the group and half to myself. They laughed because they all knew me and knew I would take on this new crusade. A new future was opening the door for me! I was going to take on state politics!

On a cold, rainy night a few weeks later I drove north on I-95 to Baltimore and met with a man named John who was the President of the Brain Injury Association of Maryland (BIAM). He ran a school located at the top of a hill and in the darkness of night it looked a little like the wizard school called Hogwarts in J. K. Rowling's book Harry Potter, which had just been released. I wondered if John could cast some kind of magical spell to help with our state's problems in serving people with brain injuries.

"I want to understand why the BIAM did not push the state government to apply for a HRSA-funded TBI grant," I said when he led me to his office. We sat in two leather chairs and I watched the rain out the window as we talked. It was getting very late and I wondered if this was worth it to come all the way to Baltimore late at night when I always got lost driving in that city. Was this me chasing windmills again?

I already knew that John's wife had a brain injury and was happy when he said he completely agreed with me that we needed to do something. I didn't have to convince him because he was frustrated on a personal basis like I was. But one of the problems I learned about that night was that there was a lot of friction between the state's Department of Health and Mental Hygiene (DHMH), the state agency responsible for services to people with brain injuries, and the BIAM. It had to do with a class action law suit against the DHMH on behalf of a group of adults with brain injuries.

The next week I once again drove to Baltimore to meet with the administrators for the DHMH, John, and a few other leaders of the BIAM. We sat around a big conference table in the offices of the DHMH. After some discussion of the state's priorities, problems, and budget restrictions, we all agreed to submit a grant proposal from the DHMH with the BIAM as a subcontractor for the next round of grants from the TBI Act funding.

"Who could we get to be the Project Director?" the agency director asked. All heads turned and looked at me and I smiled. Of course I wanted to do it! I nodded and said I would be honored to do it. We shook hands and left, and I drove home anxious to tell Ed about my newest possible job.

"Are you sure you want to get involved in state politics?" Ed asked me.

"I don't know," I said. "But I want to help and right now this is the job I have."

We got the grant and in August, 1998, I became the Project Director for a new state planning project in Maryland for TBI. Maybe, I thought, I couldn't save Jeff, or salvage the TBI program at GW, but perhaps I could save the state of Maryland! In the long run, I hoped improving the state's programs for TBI would help Jeff, our family, and others like us.

The grant provided me with a small office in the same place that the BIAM offices were located, at the Kernan Hospital in Baltimore, and I began by hiring a small project staff, holding meetings with an advisory board appointed by the Governor, and conducting a statewide assessment of needs for people living in Maryland who had a brain injury or a family member with a brain injury. We did a lot that year that I was proud of, including publishing the first TBI resource directory for the state. Through a lot of meetings and discussions we created an Action Plan for the Maryland government agencies to work together to improve the system of service delivery for people with brain injuries and their families. And I got to know people working in other states doing the same kinds of projects.

The best part of that job was meeting so many people around the state and talking to brain injury survivors and their family members. At one of our town meetings I sat with a group of family members to put together a list of their priorities. They lived in a rural area and there were not enough professional services near them so they were left on their own trying to figure out how to go on with their lives after experiencing difficulties very similar to what I'd been through. They were angry.

"He just sits and watches TV all day," one mother said. "He needs something to do but he can't do much." She was in tears.

My Administrative Assistant was taking notes and she told me later she was shocked and angry when one of the mothers said about her adult child with a TBI, "I wish he hadn't lived. It would have been better if they hadn't saved him."

"How can she say that about her own son?" she asked me in private.

"Don't judge them," I told her. "They have tough problems to deal with and she's just depressed." I felt strongly that it was our job to help these people and not criticize them.

Then I met with groups of adults with brain injuries to hear their concerns and needs. They painted a different picture from what their family members described.

"I want sex," some of them said bluntly. Or "I want to get married." That made sense to me because I worried that was exactly what Jeff wanted more than a job or a college degree.

Families of people with young school-aged children showed up for the town meetings sometimes, and it was obvious that the schools were struggling to help them and their families. Teachers and administrators did not understand TBI. But I saw that at least those families had some support from the schools and other community organizations; their kids were growing and developing so they had hope that they could change the situation. It was the families of brain-injured adults who seemed the most stressed and worried about the future. In some cases, they expressed no hope for anything better.

Meeting those families at town meetings or focus groups was sometimes like looking into a mirror. Besides feeling energized that I could help change things for these people, I was encouraged to see from talking to them that I was not imagining how difficult my life was. Sometimes that validation was just what I needed at the time because of the ups and downs at home and the fact that there were days I felt Jeff would never be able to get it all together. When I saw people who had worse situations than us it also reminded me to be happy that Jeff survived his car crash and that he was doing as well as he was, well enough to be out in the world causing chaos. And when I talked with Jeff or his friends about the work we were doing they all thanked me and were full of ideas and suggestions that seemed to make them feel involved. My personal life and professional life were seamless now and whether that was a good thing, or not, I did not know. What I did know was that it was draining and hard for me to be objective about the work

My job running that first Maryland state TBI project and trying to create systemic change in our state was not just a job to me. It was another intense crusade I was on, and an emotional roller coaster. Sometimes I came home from the meetings and had to spend a day or two recuperating and crying. I tried to focus on the positive impact this would all have in the long run. The hardest part was the state advisory meetings when I saw people I knew could do more sitting back and hiding behind their titles, not saying anything. I spent a lot of time meeting with government leaders privately so they could be open and not worry about how they made their agency or someone else look in a meeting. And finally we came up with a statewide action plan and developed subcommittees to work on each aspect of that plan. I was proud of the work we did and of my part in it.

At the end of that state planning grant period I worked with the BIAM and DHMH to write another grant proposal. When Maryland received the grant funding for their second TBI project, Ed and I talked about the wisdom of me staying on as Project Director again. He cautioned me that I might want to get the project started and then find something else to do because it was beginning to be politically difficult. People on my various committees were arguing with each other, with me, and with the leaders of both the DHMH and the state brain injury association. I felt that power struggles were starting as people saw opportunities for new jobs or funding for their agencies and organizations from the work we were doing.

I was taken by surprise not long after we received the second grant when the Chair of the Board and the Executive Director of the BIAM came to my office and told me to leave, dismissing me from the project that I had led them to get funding for. After a few days I learned that their decision was not really about me but more about the ongoing conflicts between the BIAM and DHMH in their roles as advocates versus the bureaucrats. I was caught in the cross fire, but I was still deeply hurt. It had been my personal crusade after all. Or had it?

I cried on Ed's shoulder for days, asking him "What am I going to do now?"

"Just remember this was never what you really wanted to do. It was a part of your journey and not your destination," he said trying to comfort me like he always did. "You will land where you are meant to be."

For a few weeks after I left and word got out, people would call me whispering about what they thought happened, and sending email notes telling me bits of information about something they knew that would explain it. I decided that if I could see a positive side to this experience it was that I had "arrived" because I was the target of a political coup, which made me laugh.

And it wasn't long before my own problems had to take a back seat to Jeff's.

I still had my hopes that Jeff would someday be on his own and able to hold down a job and maybe get married. But the reality for the moment was that he had no clear path to do that. Jeff had lost another job and was depressed, but I had no idea how severely because he didn't tell me, and maybe because I was involved with my own woes.

I knew some things were not going well for him because I had been trying to help him get out of trouble. A few months earlier he was acting strange and left a contract lying around in the kitchen. It was for a business managing vending machines that Jeff and a friend had decided to start together. The friend had a brain injury, was blind, and there was no way the two of them could do what they said they would do. I saw in the contract that they had promised to pay $30,000 to start this business. Say, what? I picked up the phone and called the number on the contract.

"Do you know that one of your recruiters has signed a contract with two guys who have severe brain injuries?" I asked the woman who answered the phone. "It's probably illegal because one of them is also blind and I think not even his own legal guardian."

She agreed it was wrong and wisely let them out of the contract.

After that confusion, and once Jeff got over being angry that I had stopped his brilliant business venture, he once again went through numerous short-term sales jobs, some lasting only a day or two, and now here he was unemployed again. He was also upset because he and Mimi broke up, and Jeff was still hanging on to the relationship trying to stay friends with her. I figured he would find someone else like he always did and that eventually we would get him into a job that worked for him. I was used to Jeff's employment ups and downs.

Not long after leaving the Maryland TBI project, I came home to find a note on the table from Jeff saying he was a disappointment to everyone and he was going to kill himself. I read that note and went into hysterics, my heart sinking as I realized how unhappy he had been. Now he was gone in his old Chrysler and I had no idea where he was or what to do.

I called Jeff's neuropsychologist crying into the phone and explaining what had happened. He told me to call the police. The officer who came to our house to take the report turned out to be someone Jeff knew in high school and she remembered his car accident and understood when I explained the situation. She put out an All-Points Bulletin (APB) and I sat at home waiting and continuing to cry and pace the floor.

Ed came home from work and we both waited by the phone until about eight o'clock that evening when the police called to say Jeff had been stopped in Delaware and was being detained until we got there. Ed and I just looked at each other in confusion.

Delaware? I didn't know what he was doing there but we jumped into the car and drove to a gas station on Interstate 95 to pick him up. Jeff came to the car looking sheepish and thanked us for driving all the way up there to get him. By that time Ed and I were alternating between being angry and laughing, partly out of relief that he looked okay and partly because this was just another episode in our crazy life with Jeff.

The highway patrol officer who was waiting with Jeff told us they had been stopped because the car was weaving and he and his partner thought they had a drunk driver. When they checked the license plates and saw the APB they got in touch with us. It turned out Jeff was with his buddy, Rob, who had a brain injury and no driver's license, and he had let Rob drive so he could nap a little. Rob was one of Jeff's friends with such a severe TBI and memory impairment that he would call the house and then a minute later call again insisting he had never called before that.

It was fortunate they weren't killed. That fact did not escape me, but I was very confused about what was going on with Jeff. I drove Jeff home in my car and Ed drove Rob back in Jeff's car, and on the way I tried to get more of the story.

"Jeff, what were you doing driving to Delaware?" I asked him. After spending all evening on an emotional roller coaster, I was now pissed. He looked at me in confusion as if he didn't understand why I was angry.

"You left me a suicide note, remember?"

He was surprised. "I did? Gee Mom, I'm sorry." He said he did not remember at all that he had left the note and that he was planning to kill himself.

"I think I was depressed so I called Rob," he said.

As bits of the story unfolded I learned that Rob, being a good impulsive TBI friend, told Jeff to come to his house, so Jeff just put the note on the table and forgot about it. When he got to the house, they talked and then Rob said, "Hey man! Let's go to Philly and get a hoagie!" Never mind that Philadelphia was a four-hour drive, off they went, heading north on the crowded Interstate 95 highway to get a sandwich. By that time suicide was not even a thought.

Meanwhile I was at home going crazy, and the police were searching for him? This could not continue. As we talked on the way home, I questioned Jeff about why he had been so depressed and I was so engrossed in the conversation that I did not even realize it when I hit a dead deer on the winding roads of the more rural part of Silver Spring, Maryland. I felt the car bump into something and sail through the air, but I just kept going. The next day Ed took it to a mechanic and they said there was deer blood on the bottom of the car.

I had to help Jeff get his life together, partly because his life and mine were so intertwined that I knew I couldn't stand much more of this. I was trying so hard to be supportive of him and I felt like he wasn't doing his part, which I also knew wasn't fair because he was trying. While Ed was at the mechanic's shop, I began an all-out renewed effort to help Jeff plan his life better and to figure out what kind of employment he could maintain so that he could move out of the house like he said he wanted to. I needed for him to get out on his own.

"You need a job," I said for the umpteenth thousandth time. "And you get bored with just any old job so you need a real career. We are going to find something!"

I went to the bookshelves and pulled out self-help books I had that included career and interest tests, and we talked about what he could do. I was convinced that his depression had to do with not having a job he could support himself with, and I tried to reassure him that he was still a smart person and that we would help him figure out what to do with his life.

"Well, I was thinking maybe I could become a teacher," he said.

Jeff as a classroom teacher might have been good years ago but didn't seem like a good fit now with his memory problems. I needed to shift him to something else.

"Maybe. But what do you enjoy doing the most, when you have free time?" I asked him.

He thought for a minute. "Well, I always like to play computer games," he said.

Okay, now we were onto something! Travis was home and he chimed in saying that in high school Jeff was a very good programmer and had made As in programming classes. I'd forgotten that. When Ed got home we were all still engrossed in this latest fixing Jeff conversation, and his eyes lit up because he was a computer programmer and he said he could help Jeff with this. Ed loved being useful.

Yes! We had a solution! Jeff would become a computer programmer. We signed him up for a trade school called Computer Learning Center (CLC) and Jeff and I met with a new DORS counselor. The counselor said that they would pay for his tuition, and help him find a job when he graduated in about six months. I thought this would work better than trying to take college classes because the program at CLC was in modules and very structured and concrete. After paying for college classes that he failed, I was learning that Jeff had trouble fitting in on a college campus and with the many distractions there. At CLC I thought he would not have that problem. The students were mostly guys about his age and it was located in a small facility in the back of a shopping center and not a campus.

Jeff did well with his CLC classes and passed through the first two modules with all As. The plan was that he would graduate after he finished the third. Travis had graduated by that time from the University of Maryland with his degree in Civil Engineering, led the senior class project, and now had his first engineering job.

We all cheered when Jeff told us CLC was having a graduation ceremony in Columbia, Maryland and Travis even got off work early to join us for the ceremony. I thought it was a little unusual to have a graduation ceremony at a restaurant but we dressed up and drove the forty five minutes to Columbia with Jeff beaming the entire way there.

When we got to the restaurant, we walked in and told the host we were there for the CLC graduation. He looked confused and checked the schedule, and shook his head. Oh no, I thought; this is not what we thought it was. But what is it?

"I'm sorry but we have nothing like that," the host said. Jeff looked embarrassed and stepped forward taking charge.

"I made a reservation for Bouck," he said. "For four."

The host checked his reservation list, nodded, and someone else appeared saying to follow her.

I was beginning to feel a little nauseated as we walked behind Jeff to a table, and sat down waiting for him to explain. In my peripheral vision I could see Travis and Ed becoming angry. I wanted to stay calm until we heard what Jeff had to say, but it was not easy considering how many times we had been misled before.

Jeff began to tell us that no, there was no graduation but he had big news, and Travis interrupted him.

"Jeff, this is bullshit!" he said. "I took off work for this?" He got up and walked out.

I couldn't blame Travis for his outburst but I only felt hollow inside, and sad, and I put my hand on Ed's under the table to ask him not to say what I knew he wanted to say. I knew how much Ed hated lying, maybe even more than I did.

Jeff explained, as if it was all perfectly logical and reasonable, that he had quit CLC about two months earlier but he had a great job he was excited about. His eyes were dancing as if he was high on drugs, but I knew it was just another TBI moment, or at least I thought that was all it was.

"So where have you been going every day?" I asked quietly.

"So you're not graduating?" Ed asked. He was now glaring at Jeff who seemed surprised that we saw this as a problem.

"I thought when I told you about my new job it wouldn't matter," he said defensively. He pulled out information about the company he had signed up with and it did look interesting. They were a new group of programmers and it might be a good idea except that the office was almost a two-hour drive from our house.

He explained that he had not been going to classes for a while, and no, he was not graduating. However he did finish the first two modules and that was enough because he had found this great job in Virginia. No problem, see? His eyes implored me to be proud of him and I tried but all I felt was that he was missing the point.

I went back to my other question he had not yet answered.

"Like I said, Jeff, where have you been going every day when we thought you were in school?"

It turned out he had become involved with a woman he met somewhere near the CLC school building, and that was why he quit school. He was kicked out for not attending classes and lost the financial support from DORS. In fact he now owed them money to pay for classes he never completed.

Jeff started his job the next week, convinced this would all work out and he would be rich and successful. He left home very early in the mornings to drive around the Beltway and through what was commonly referred to as the mixing bowl, into northern Virginia, and out to the suburbs where the office was located. He would get home at seven or eight at night completely exhausted and obviously frustrated. The job lasted about two months. Predictably, because it was such a long commute, he was frequently late for work and he could not keep up with the rapid pace of a growing technology consulting company.

He went back to a state of depression, sleeping all day and not showering or shaving. I saw a pattern beginning to emerge. Jeff would get something like a new job, or register for school; then he would find a woman he was excited about, get involved with her, lose the job or fail classes, and then get seriously depressed. He would quickly go from thinking he could handle anything and everything to feeling hopeless and worthless.

Through his professional connections Ed found Jeff another computer programming job closer to home, and we decided this time we needed to be more involved. This job was with a government contract agency large enough to offer him some support as a new programmer and with a salary that had real potential to give him the independence he wanted.

I set up an appointment with the organization that years before had provided Jeff with his outpatient rehabilitation services, and they set him up with a job coach who said he would meet with Jeff and his employer on a regular basis. The young man, Trevor, was a nice, hip-looking guy with a ponytail but Jeff didn't like him and quickly began to lie to him like he did to me.

"Jeff, we are all on your team," I told him when Trevor met with all of us at our house. "We just want to make sure you are clear about what's expected of you. And if you have any problems, like you did in other jobs, Trevor will be there to help you problem-solve." Jeff nodded and said he understood.

Then Trevor called me one evening to tell me Jeff was missing work and not showing up on time. We set up an on-site meeting at Jeff's workplace with Jeff, Trevor, Ed and me, and Jeff's immediate supervisor.

"He's a good programmer," his supervisor said. "But he misinterprets instructions sometimes. And he needs things repeated so often because he forgets, and we can't always do that."

We discussed strategies that we thought might help him.

"The real problem though," she said, "is that he has frequent absences and comes in late, and he doesn't communicate with us about it. We have a flexible schedule and he can change his hours but he has to work it out with us."

We left the meeting with a written plan and Jeff promised to be more open with people about the problems he was having with keeping up. I thought the flexible schedule was not a good idea for someone like Jeff but he insisted it was not the problem.

Shortly after that meeting Trevor called me.

"I'm sorry but I can't work with Jeff anymore because of his lying," he said. "There are things you don't know and I don't want to be in the middle."

I didn't know what he meant by things we did not know, but I told Trevor I understood and that I knew he had tried. At the same time as Jeff was struggling to keep up with his new computer programming job, he began dating a girl named Heather.

When we first met Heather, Jeff said she was just a friend and was there at our house because she was dating his friend Bobby who was coming over later. It wasn't long, however, before she began showing up at our house alone with Jeff and not with Bobby or any of his other friends, and it seemed obvious to me that they were becoming a couple.

"Are you involved with Heather?" I asked him. With Jeff I knew I had to be direct because otherwise he would keep important information from me until he found himself in over his head. He thought he could handle things he couldn't, things I knew he was not ready for because of his brain injury.

"No, not really. We're just friends, and besides she isn't my type."

I didn't know if he was lying to me or himself. But lying to others, for all of us, does usually start with those things we all do to block the truth from ourselves when we know people won't like it, or when it's embarrassing, or when we don't accept that part of ourselves. I realized that was normal human fallacy, but it was made worse by Jeff's brain injury; there was so much he forgot or didn't know about himself.

Ed and I were sitting on the sofa in our family room watching TV when Jeff walked in and asked to talk to us. We turned off the TV and braced ourselves for whatever he had to say, having been through enough bizarre episodes of the soap opera I call "Life with Jeff and his TBI" to expect anything.

I did not see this one coming though. He held up his left hand and stood there in front of us waiting for it to sink in. On his finger was a wedding ring.

"Huh? You're married?" I asked in shock. "When? Who? Why?"

"Heather. A month ago," he said, tilting his chin up in that defiant way he has when he's done something he knows I think is stupid but he's pleased with himself because it was an act of independence and asserting himself. Since his TBI, my son's driving motivation had been a desire to reclaim his independence and I knew that. But my thinking was: why this? How was marrying Heather, who even he knew was all wrong for him, a step toward independence?

As I let Jeff's news sink in, the shock wore off a little so that a new realization slowly hit my conscious thoughts. He had been married and yet living at our house like always for a month, like nothing had changed, as if he was still the same single Jeff looking for love in all the wrong places.

I could feel Ed next to me about to explode in rage and I myself was getting dizzy and sick to my stomach. This was not the first time Jeff had deceived us, but I felt it might be the biggest. I began to cry at the enormity and permanency of this newest bad decision he had made. This definitely was not in The Plan; this was all Jeff's Plan. He had made some crazy choices in his life before, but this was a doozy.

Jeff told us the story of how he and this girl we barely knew, someone he had told me he was not attracted to but who I had seen hanging around way too much, got married at a courthouse and then spent two nights at a hotel for their "honeymoon." That was when he was declared AWOL from his job and fired.

Now I understood a lot of things that had been going on, recent times that had not made sense and that had been keeping me awake at night trying to figure it out. This was the missing piece of the puzzle and the reason Jeff had been acting so secretive and why he mysteriously lost the perfectly good job as a computer programmer that was part of The Plan, the master plan to get a good job that would give him an income he could live on. This was probably what Trevor was referring to that led to him resigning as Jeff's job coach.

Then another thought hit me: where was Heather?

"Where is she?" I asked.

"She's at home," he said. Still looking sheepish, he explained that she went back to live with her mother and he came home to our house, back to his old bedroom, because they had no jobs and nowhere to live. Oh no, I thought, here it comes. He is in over his head again and Ed and I will have to bail him out.

I began to cry and yell at him.

"Jeff, how could you get married and not even tell me? What the hell are you going to do?" I screamed, and then another awful thought hit me. I held my breath as I asked him, "Is she pregnant?"

"No," he laughed. I saw nothing funny here.

"Well, that makes eloping all the more ridiculous!" I said. He began to look regretful and I went from anger to sadness. I could see reality slowly creeping into Jeff's brain like the awareness a tornado is coming. His neuropsychologist once said Jeff only has two weather reports for his moods: skies extremely sunny and skies extremely dark. Storm clouds were gathering in his face.

"Jeff, if you really wanted to get married, I wanted to be there to dance at your wedding." I began to cry, sad that after all we had been through together Jeff cut me out of such an important event in his life.

We all needed to just talk, so I tried to calm down. Ed and I reminded Jeff that we were both on his team and that's why we had been working with his neuropsychologist and job coach to help him get that good job and keep it so that he had an income. We were his family and we were all trying to help him gain his independence and move into an apartment on his own like he said he wanted to. If he wanted to get married and have a family, the plan had been that he would be able to do it, but he had no job so this was all backwards; didn't he see that?

He looked crushed and defeated as he listened and seemed to understand what he had done. "I'm sorry Mom," he said in all sincerity. "It was her idea."

I dissolved into more tears.

With all my heart I loved this messed up guy standing in front of us looking so miserable. But the predicaments he got himself into were an ongoing problem for Ed and me and at that moment I felt like my head was going to explode from the frustration I felt.

"Jeff, what are you two planning to do? Where are you going to live and how will you support yourselves?" Even as I asked the questions I knew it was unreasonable for me to expect anything else. His frontal lobe damage was the reason for it all.

He looked thoughtful and then said what I had been dreading. For now, just until they got on their feet, and got jobs, could they please just live with us? So that was their plan? Depend on us, our house, and our money; that was it?

Ed and I looked at each other in dismay and I knew what he was thinking. Ed did not like Heather and did not trust her, and he did not want her moving into our house. But what choice did we have? I mentally ran through our options starting with maybe I could declare this marriage to be a sign of his mental incompetence and have it annulled. I knew I couldn't do that without a legal battle though because I was not legal guardian for Jeff.

This was not the first time I regretted that I never got legal guardianship after his brain injury, which several people advised me to do. One person who was adamant about it was the director of the day program Jeff attended because she had a daughter with a TBI who had become involved in some serious trouble and she was able to help her only because she did have that legal right. Jeff was over eighteen so legally he could make his own stupid and even dangerous decisions. But I didn't do it because I knew Jeff so well and how important independence was to him, and that he was terrified I would take away his freedom. Just the mention of guardianship always sent him into a fit of anger and rebellion, and he even ran away for two days one time because I threatened it.

Ed and I went upstairs to our bedroom and shut the door to talk. We discussed saying no; they could not live with us. But where would they go and how would they manage? I was afraid they would be on the streets or living in a homeless shelter and that scared me even more than having them in our basement. In the end we told Jeff yes they could stay at our house for a few months, until they got jobs, but they had to find jobs, sign a rental agreement, pay rent and help around the house. He said they would do all of that, of course, and he thanked us.

The next day the doorbell rang and I opened it to find my new daughter-in-law standing on our porch with her purse and no suitcase. I wondered: where were her things? But I didn't ask and just hugged her instead.

"Welcome to the family," I told her, trying to be a good mother-in-law. She giggled.

The next day I took her out to lunch to get to know her better and she told me about her family and her background, and I felt a new surge of compassion for her. She grew up in poverty and I wanted to help her as much as I could. I convinced Ed we should take her out to buy her clothes because she had so little, and he agreed to it to keep me happy. We had fun that day and I felt good about the efforts we were making to treat her like family and accept their marriage. Seeing how happy Jeff was, I had new hopes that with our help they could become more independent and this would all turn out for the best. Maybe with a wife to support Jeff would be more motivated to get a job and keep it.

I was worried but still tried to be hopeful that, in spite of this new wrinkle in our plan, Jeff could hold down a responsible job. But I was baffled because, even though it was obvious that the expectations of a company doing computer programming were possibly too hard for him, he did have help and I thought he could have learned and been successful over time. He needed to use compensatory strategies like a job coach, a note taker in meetings, and memory aids; all of which we had tried to provide for him.

"I think it's more than his brain injury," I told Ed when we talked about it. "Some of my graduate students have had a TBI just as severe as Jeff's and they can stay focused and use disability resources and strategies to do a lot more than him. It may take longer to learn than for other people, but he should be able to do this."

"We can't help him if he's going to lie to us," Ed said and I knew that was true.

Jeff had done his usual good job of lying to all of us to cover up the fact that he was married and that this relationship was too much for him to handle along with work. Before we knew about the elopement, after he was fired from the latest job, we had a series of conversations about what Jeff wanted in life, the kind of thing I always became fixated on with him, but those conversations with Jeff usually went nowhere because he didn't follow up on whatever great ideas we planned.

"Jeff, if I'm working harder on your life than you are, I think I am the one who has a problem," I said. "I need to stop doing that."

Even Jeff agreed.

"I just need for you to promise me you will ask for help, from me or someone, when you need help. I can't let go of trying to help you if I don't know you have someone. You understand?"

He nodded but I wasn't sure he would remember and do what I was asking him to do. And so I said I was going to stop trying to fix Jeff's problems, but inside I knew that I could not let go of that role until I saw evidence that he was taking better care of himself. His car crash was still too fresh in my memory, and maybe it always will be.

And now he had a wife. And they lived in our basement.

The months went by; they found part-time jobs, they lost the jobs, they found others, lost them, and they never paid a penny of the rent they said they would pay. Jeff helped now and then with picking things up or clearing the table but Heather never did, and the basement apartment we provided for them was a disgusting mess of dirty clothes, candy wrappers, and pizza boxes. Ed and I were both working long hours and were becoming increasingly enraged. We watched them come and go with their friends like two teenagers without a care in the world and Ed said he felt used, but when I tried talking to Jeff about it he reacted by getting angry with me.

"We know you don't want us here and we plan to move out soon!" he said. "Heather found an apartment we can afford!" But of course I knew it was a fantasy; they couldn't afford anything. I didn't know what to do.

I was in my home office on the first floor of our house one day when Heather came in and stood at my elbow as I tried to work. I looked up at her and waited to hear what she had to say.

"Jeff isn't managing money very well," she said in her little girl voice. Sometimes she was loud and aggressive and at other times sounded like a child. I had come to understand that it depended on what she wanted. She had an act for every occasion.

"Well, you two do have serious money problems and you need to figure it out. Talk to him," I said. Her face fell and she ran downstairs to the basement. The next thing I knew Jeff was home from work yelling at me because Heather had called him crying and said I was being mean to her.

"Jeff, that's not true," I said, trying to stay calm and not to escalate the situation. "Where is she? Let's talk about this." But he shook his head and disappeared.

I looked out the front window to see her meeting him in the front yard and realized she had gone out the patio door from the basement and around the house to avoid me. I could see her waving her arms and yelling, him glancing at the house in a rage, and then they got in the car and left. Dramas like that kept happening.

Ed became so angry about the situation that he was up at night every night, pacing and acting like a raving lunatic, and we argued all the time about it. Ed said she was taking advantage of Jeff and us. I tried to convince him that we should give her a chance, that she was just young and from a different kind of family than ours. I didn't like having her there either but I thought I could talk with her and somehow make this all work out. But I hated that Ed and I were at odds and that he was so unhappy.

One of the things I always loved about Ed and our relationship was that we talked everything over for as long as it took until we felt it was resolved. For us to be angry and at an impasse like this, for the first time ever, worried me. I set up an appointment with Jeff's neuropsychologist and when we met and explained how bad things were at our house he told Ed that he should not have to live with someone he does not want to live with. Sometimes I have a hard time seeing that I am causing a problem because I like to believe that I have an endless capacity for understanding and compromise, but that day I saw that my insistence on helping Jeff no matter what was unfair to Ed. Our home was ours, his and mine, and he did not feel comfortable or even safe with Heather there.

We agreed that they needed to move out, but I was reluctant to tell them and Ed wasn't going to do it. I was not sure where they would go because they had no money to live on, and I was afraid for Jeff. I pictured things like them moving to a homeless shelter and Jeff trying to protect his wife, getting into a fight and being killed or ending up in jail. With Jeff, my mind always went to the worst possible scenario for good reasons. So, since neither Ed nor I could tell them they had to move out, we continued to let them live with us, trying to gently ease them out on their own. I did what I always did and tried to help them figure out what jobs they could get and where they could live.

Even though I could not tell them to leave, a solution was provided for us. Ed and I left them alone at the house for a few days while I was speaking at a brain injury conference in Kansas

City. We returned to find Jeff and Heather gone, the basement trashed, and a note on the kitchen table.

The note was from Heather telling me that they were moving back to western Maryland to be near her mother and sister, because it was cheaper to live there. She added that maybe she would forgive me for being so mean to her, because she was a "good Christian," and maybe she would let me see the baby.

I was going to be a grandmother! I had been envious of my friends with grandchildren for years, but this was not how I pictured it happening. Still, I was excited about a baby in the family.

Jeff showed up at the house a few days later to collect things they left behind, and we had a huge argument. To him it was a perfectly reasonable, normal decision to take his pregnant wife and start their new life in a place that was not as expensive as Montgomery County, and for her to be next to her family while they had their first baby.

Ed and I agreed that it did make sense in some ways and was better than going to a shelter like he had said they might do, but I was still afraid for him. After all, he had only lived away from home twice in his twenty-eight years of life. Once for six months when he was in the hospital and inpatient rehabilitation after his TBI, and the one year he went away to college, which was a disaster.

With frontal lobe damage to my brain it is sometimes difficult to plan for the future and, with being unable to look at the past, unless I have help from other people who know me. My career now is raising my daughter and this is a job that is the most rewarding challenge possible.

—Jeff Bouck, TBI Survivor

Chapter 9

Our Tribe Scatters

DURING THE FALL OF 2000, both of my young adult sons began following their own dreams and letting go of the family enmeshment that had come about naturally after Jeff's TBI. I think this happens to so many families after trauma. People who are by nature introverted and independent of others, like Steve, may drift apart from the family while people like me who are emotionally centered and need other people try to hang onto everyone. Anyway, whatever the reason, I wanted to keep our new family together for as long as I could. It was a pattern I was probably repeating from my childhood family. I had learned in my many years of therapy that I try too much to help other people as a way to run away from dealing with my own emotions.

There are essentially two kinds of dysfunctional families according to some authors of family systems theory, which I have taught in my classes on building family partnerships for students with brain injuries. One type is the detached family which is characterized by each family member remaining separate and independent of one another, not communicating. Detached families have a lack of connection and trust among the individuals who make up the parts of the system. Then there is the kind I grew up in, the enmeshed family, with no boundaries and too much connection. I did not have any privacy or a separate identity from my mother until I forced it in my late teens and twenties, and then I felt she was always angry with me and she said things that made me out to be a mean and ungrateful daughter. As I began to individuate, and figure out who I was separate from her, she began to act at times like she hated me; it felt I had to choose between my relationship with her and my own identity. I did not want to do that to my kids.

My sons needed to have their own lives and now they were doing that, so the educated and reasonable side of me said, "This is normal, healthy and good." But my traumatized mother self, the one who was still afraid to let go of them, was not happy with the transition process. Our tribe was scattering and I was experiencing the delayed grieving I had not fully done in 1990.

Jeff and Heather were now living in western Maryland starting their own family, and Travis and Becky were away at graduate school in Charlottesville, Virginia where Travis had been accepted to the Darden School of Business for his MBA. Jeff had what he had wanted all along; he was married with a baby on the way. Travis had what he wanted; he was on the road to financial wealth and the good life. This was what I wanted for my children, wasn't it?

"Mom, we should have been out of here long ago," Travis said when I told him I missed him and Jeff. He was right of course. Travis had lived with us until he was twenty-seven and Jeff was twenty-nine. So, after all, it wasn't like they were leaving home too young or anything.

I knew I was being ridiculous but couldn't help it so I had to do a lot of internal work in order to let go. I had to work on trusting that Jeff had his own Higher Power watching over him and would not end up in serious trouble just because I was not nearby to help and guide him. And I had to trust that Travis would keep in touch and continue to include me in his life.

"I know it's just grandiosity," I said to Ed. "I have to stop thinking that someone else's life is up to me." I journaled about it and talked about it with friends, and eventually the feelings began to fade. After a little while I began to enjoy this new phase of my life and to see that there were a lot of positives.

Ed and I were finally able to live like newlyweds alone in our house, with just each other, and we could do what we wanted to without worrying about where the kids were or when they would come home. We had sex on the sofa, went out to dinner on the spur of the moment, and we argued out in the open. If I hadn't been so worried about Jeff I would have been completely happy.

Another good part of the kids leaving home was that I felt free to focus on my work, and I spent time writing another grant proposal with Carol Kochhar at GW for funding the Master's degree program in brain injury and special education that had been dormant now for several years. My dream was still to be working at GW and in order to do that I knew I had to help get the funding because brain injury as a field was still too new for the university to fully embrace it. University professional preparation programs tend to follow the lead of the needs in the professional field they are training students for.

At that time the public, including schools and human service organizations, did not understand the need for education about brain injury. In the government it was considered a "low incidence" population and that meant there was little demand for, or funding for, professional training programs related to TBI even though there was now a special education category called Students with Traumatic Brain Injury. I knew that there were a lot more kids and adults living with TBI than people realized. There were kids who had TBIs that were never reported, those with undiagnosed TBI from concussions due to playground or sports injuries, and a lot of kids who were just not in special education so the government did not know about them. Teachers and parents so often just waited for the physical healing process and did not think about long term impact on learning, socialization, and emotional adjustment after a brain injury. A lot of the students with TBI, I had learned, were identified incorrectly as Learning Disabled (LD), Mentally Retarded (MR), Other Health Impaired (OHI), or even Emotionally/Behaviorally Disturbed (ED/BD). And I knew from working in nursing homes that a lot of older adults were misdiagnosed as having Alzheimer's Disease or other types of Dementia after a brain injury.

In the spring of 2001 I was asked to speak at a brain injury conference in Williamsburg, Virginia. My talk focused on learning theory and the neurological and cognitive changes after a TBI. I included my own observations about Jeff and our family, explaining how his TBI disrupted his ability to learn and therefore his entire life and our family dynamics. I talked about the role that schools could play in helping children with brain injuries when teachers had an understanding about how a TBI affected the learning process, and I talked about the program at GW and that I was afraid it was dying for lack of funding.

A man seated in the front row of the audience asked a lot of questions so I was not surprised when he came to talk to me afterward. He introduced himself as Greg Rooker and said he would like for me to meet his wife, Fran Rooker, who was in another room.

I had dinner that evening with the Rookers and they told me the story of their young son, Jason, who died a year after he had a brain injury from an accidental hanging in their front yard. We talked and talked, sharing the heartache that we all had with something like that happening to a child. It was a bond I had found all parents of children with brain injuries shared. And so many of us were also the ones trying to raise public awareness and educate people about the effects of a TBI.

"How much would you need to get the program started up again?" Greg asked me.

I hadn't thought about it but quoted an amount off the top of my head, estimating funds for student tuition stipends and some administrative costs for at least a year.

"We want to help," he said. "We have set up a foundation in Jason's name called the Jason Foundation." After that night we continued to talk on the phone and by email, and I met with them and people from GW to work it all out. During the fall of 2001, the Jason Foundation provided generous funding to GW and soon after that Carol and I received word that the federal grant proposal we had submitted was also approved. It was all happening. I would be going back to work at GW full time now, to do the work I had wanted to do for ten years.

Meeting the Rookers changed my life, and it was another reminder to me that all I need to do is say what I need. I will be forever grateful to them.

I began interviewing prospective new students for the program, developing new courses, going to faculty meetings, and talking to people on campus about all of the other ideas I had been thinking about for years and finally had the chance to implement. I could not wait to build the brain injury training program beyond what it had been to what I thought it needed to be. I felt alive and on fire again and I loved it.

With the help of Carol and the university's development office, I established a new Center on Education and Human Services in Acquired Brain Injury at GW to combine teaching classes with research, and I continued writing more grant proposals for more funding. Then I developed a graduate certificate program in brain injury and put the courses online so that people living in other locations could learn about the impact of a TBI on survivors and their families, and develop the skills to help them.

Travis graduated in May that year and he and Becky were married in June in a beautiful destination wedding on a Caribbean island. Steve and his mother were there along with Becky's family, Ed and me, and a few of their old friends. We had fun all week, staying in a villa on top of a cliff overlooking the ocean, and spending time with people celebrating the beginning of my son's marriage. I even enjoyed seeing Steve and reconnecting with his mother, whom I had maintained a positive but somewhat distant relationship with over the years.

The only blight on an otherwise wonderful experience was that Jeff was supposed to be his brother's best man and he wasn't there. Heather would not allow him to go to the wedding, which enraged Travis and Ed and saddened me. When Jeff told Travis, a few weeks earlier, that he would not be there Travis said they had a big row on the phone.

"She's only going to be your wife for a few years and I'm going to be your brother for the rest of your life!" Travis said he told him. Harsh but probably true. Jeff hung up on him and they didn't speak after that.

When Travis and Becky returned from their honeymoon, they moved into our basement for a few months until they found a house to buy. They were ideal tenants, helping around the house and even repainting the basement for us and we all got along well. Despite all of the trauma and upheavals in our life I now saw us going through a normal process of all of us moving on, my life going in new directions I could never have imagined in 1989. I was happy with my marriage to Ed; I had my Ph.D.; I was now a university professor; my sons were both married; and soon I would be a grandmother.

How did this all happen so fast? It seemed like it had only been a few years since I was lost career-wise, afraid of being all alone without ever finishing my Ph.D., struggling with my divorce from Steve, and coping with the aftermath of Jeff's car accident and a rebellious teenage Travis. At that time I never would have believed how much our family and my life could change in just ten years.

In the fall of 2001 I walked into my classroom for the first Introduction to Acquired Brain Injury course in the new program I was developing. A room full of new students stood up and applauded. What a feeling that was; not only was I able to do the work I wanted to do but I had found students who believed, as I did, that this program had been worth saving. They were all crusaders like me.

Even though my work was heading in the direction I wanted, I was frantic with worry about Jeff and the baby who was on the way. I could not imagine how Jeff and Heather would be able to take care of a baby when they seemed so unable to take care of themselves.

One day I was in my office when a young woman came to see me. She was still in an undergraduate program in another state but was interested in applying to our Master's degree program when she finished her degree, and she told me her passion for brain injury came from having a father with a TBI. She said he had been her stay-at-home parent all of her life while her mother worked.

I told her about Jeff and how worried I was about the baby.

"The baby will be okay," she said. I cried and hugged her.

She was like an angel who appeared in my life at just the right time. I was learning that accepting reality was the key to happiness and peace. We couldn't do anything to help Jeff because it was his decision to elope, to move away, and to allow his wife to block our phone calls and demand that he not communicate with us. I had made mistakes in my life, so why couldn't he? My job was just to be there for him when it all fell apart.

I decided Jeff was entitled to the same misery as anyone else stuck in a bad marriage and who just didn't know it yet. He needed respect for his autonomy, something all young adults crave and something that he had been robbed of. Because he had a disability did not mean I should take over his life and not give him the chance to learn from his mistakes.

I went back to praying to that God I still was not sure I believed in because now it was not just about my son with a brain injury. There was an innocent child now about to be born into the world; a baby I was afraid would have to suffer if Jeff didn't handle his life better than he had in the past. Knowing Jeff as I did, I knew he would never want that to happen. I put him and the baby in a God Box.

Then on September 11, 2001 terrorists attacked on our country and once again the future became uncertain.

That morning I was at a board meeting for Brain Injury Services (BIS), the case management company I was involved with, when the receptionist pulled us all out of the meeting to watch what was happening on a small television they had in the front office. I could not believe my eyes as I watched it happening from the BIS offices about a mile away from the Pentagon, and my first thought was of people I knew who worked there. My next thought was of Becky because she was at home alone and I did not want her to see the news and be afraid. Our house was clear around the Beltway and it would take at least an hour to get home. Like other busy people in the DC area, our family was scattered all over the place.

Ed was at work in downtown Washington DC, Travis was at a training session for his new consulting job a few blocks from the White House, I was in Virginia, and Becky was in our house in Maryland by herself. Jeff was now living three hours away, near where another plane crashed as passengers tried to stop the terrorists as I learned later. I was in a panic as I drove home. I called Becky and Ed briefly but my cell phone was cut off while I was talking to him. I found out from listening to my car radio that the government had stopped all cell service in the Washington DC area for national security purposes.

It took Ed and Travis a long time to get home on the metro that day, but eventually we were all together huddled in our basement watching the terrible events of the day. The next week was a nightmare for everyone, and classes at GW were cancelled because the university is a short distance from both the White House and the State Department. When classes resumed we had constant bomb threats and buildings were heavily guarded.

"Ed, I wonder if we should move away from DC," I said one night when I was doing my usual thing of trying to predict the future.

"But this will all settle down eventually, and our jobs and everything are here," he said. He was right of course. I loved so much about living in the DC area including our house and my job. I wanted to be at GW until I was too old to manage the streets of DC or climb the stairs in the university buildings, and I wanted to keep doing all of the professional work I was doing to solve problems for people with brain injuries and other disabilities. This crazy DC metropolitan area was home, so I put aside the idea of moving for now. I no longer felt safe there, however, and the idea of leaving DC lurked in the back of my mind like the way the noise of an air conditioner or heater does when you are used to it and don't notice anymore.

In October, 2001, Travis and Becky moved out of our basement to their new home a few miles away, and unlike the way Jeff moved out this felt like a normal step for them and all of us.

We were all together at their new home for Thanksgiving dinner when Steve called me to say the baby was on the way. He had gone to be with Jeff and drive him to the teaching hospital in Morgantown, West Virginia where the doctor had sent Heather for the delivery. Apparently Heather allowed her mother to ride with her in the ambulance and left Jeff behind.

The next day Steve called to tell me that our granddaughter, Hannah, had been born almost two months early and weighed only four pounds, but she was healthy and doing fine.

"She's tiny but she has all of her parts," he said. "And she's just beautiful; you will love her."

I felt such a mixture of emotions: joy that I had a grandchild, relief that she was healthy, but also anger and confusion. Why was Steve the one with them for this important occasion? Why not me? I found out later that there was a simple, predictable explanation: Steve was giving them money.

Over the next month, Steve called to give me updates and I thanked him for keeping me informed. I also reminded him that supporting them was probably a mistake because he was enabling them.

"I know that," he said. "I've decided to stop giving them money and I've been meaning to tell you, I'm moving to Florida to help Mom."

I got off the phone that day and turned to Ed, laughing, to tell him the good news.

"Just wait," I said. "Now we'll hear from them."

Sure enough, about two weeks later, as soon as Steve left for Florida, the phone rang and it was Heather.

"Hi," she said as if nothing had happened, as if they hadn't blocked our calls and refused to talk to us for almost a year. "Do you want to see the baby?"

I had been practicing for this moment and jumped at it.

"Of course!" I told her. "We'll come this weekend!"

When we got to their door and knocked Heather answered holding tiny infant Hannah and handed the baby to me right away. My granddaughter was in my arms at last, dressed in a small frock with a ribbon and bow around her head. Her round, trusting infant eyes stared up at me. I fell in love instantly.

"She may need her diaper changed," Heather said with a smirk.

I nodded and took the diaper and the baby to the changing table, and then sat on the sofa and fed her a bottle that Jeff handed to me. We stayed for the weekend and I watched my son take such good care of his daughter that it brought tears of joy to my eyes. This was what he had wanted all along, not a career like I had assumed. He was the most devoted father I had ever seen. Ed and I both noticed that when Hannah cried she looked to her daddy, not her mother, and held out her arms to him. Jeff was so proud of his little family and their tiny, run-down house that he had painted himself. How could I not be happy for him after all he'd been through?

We spent the night at a small hotel near them because there was no place for us to sleep at their house. On Sunday we got to take care of Hannah and I did piles of dirty dishes, and then we took them to a laundromat where we did thirteen loads of laundry. Everything they owned seemed to be dirty. Despite the obvious mess they lived in, Ed and I made it a point to say nothing negative and to just be helpful because we wanted to make sure we could visit again.

What worried me the most was that after she handed the baby to me, I never again saw Heather pick up Hannah or care for her even when Hannah cried. After that first visit Ed and I made sure we visited them at least every two or three weeks. We drove three hours each way, a total of six hours of driving over a weekend, and often it took double that time to bring them to our house on Friday and then take them home on Sunday, but Ed and I agreed that it was worth it. As much as I did love my work at GW and enjoyed spending time with Travis and Becky, the best moments for me that year were when Hannah was with us on weekends.

I began to fix up a baby room down the hall, across from Jeff's old bedroom, which was now a guest room, so that Hannah would have her own room when they came to visit. I got a rocking chair from a friend and we bought a portable crib, and I had a ball shopping for baby clothes, stuffed animals, and educational toys. As Hannah got a little older I added a high chair in the kitchen and play things in the family room, and before long our home looked like a baby lived there.

When Hannah was with us I spent my weekends taking care of her and putting her to sleep at night because Jeff and Heather went out with friends. It wasn't long before those weekends lengthened to four or five days, with Heather going out by herself and Jeff and Hannah staying with us most of the time. Jeff seemed oblivious to the problem I saw and when I asked him about it he insisted he trusted her.

I watched as Heather began developing the relationship with Jeff's friend Barney that would eventually end their marriage. What was wrong with Jeff that he didn't see it? Would he see reality quicker than he had in the past? Oh yeah, I was forgetting all that I knew about brain injury. I understood once and for all, after so many years, that Jeff's TBI, and the cognitive effects of it, were still with him and likely to be a permanent part of him.

"Should we say anything to Jeff?" I asked Ed. My hints and questions were not working and I was thinking I should tell Jeff directly that Heather was cheating on him.

"No, he has to see it for himself," he said. I knew he was right; telling Jeff something before he saw it himself had never worked out well before.

Then I got the call from Jeff when Hannah was a little over a year old that changed all of our lives.

In 2003 I received a call from a friend that gave me what I had needed for some time; a reason to leave an abusive relationship. He told me my wife was having an affair with my so-called friend Barney. I picked up the phone, called my mother, and since then life has become nothing but better.

—Jeff Bouck, TBI Survivor

Chapter 10

Saving Hannah

IT WAS JUNE, 2003. When my thirty-one-year-old son called me from Maryland and said, "Come get us," I was clear across the country in Seattle.

What the hell, Jeff? Don't you remember where I am?

The obvious answer was: of course not. I forgot that he forgets.

I forgot because I still hadn't accepted his TBI even after fourteen years, and I fought the reality that he was so damaged. How could he not be the same child I raised, who remembered every book he'd ever read and who was able to pass his student achievement tests at the twelfth grade level when he was in eighth grade. He was a lead actor in some of our local community theater productions and school plays because he was always a quick learner, and he had so much intellectual potential that I was excited about his future. It was hard to remember that he was still smart when he did very un-smart things because of his brain injury. I didn't know why it was so hard for me to remember that, especially with all of my education.

Over the years, since Jeff's car accident in 1989, I should have learned this is the way someone living with the effects of a severe TBI often makes plans: with no forethought and with holes in the memory so that information needed for the plan to work is not included. TBI is a true One Day at a Time way of life, something I struggle with myself. I am a worrier and I live in the wreckage of the future.

I laid back against the pillows propped up on the hotel bed to talk to Jeff, and glanced at Ed with an oh no, here we go again look. Ed lounged on his side next to me and watched, waiting to hear what was going on this time.

"Jeff, we are in Seattle, remember?" I said, taking a breath and trying not to let my frustration show in my voice. I was worried about him and even more worried about the baby, so I wanted him to keep talking to me. "We'll be back tomorrow night."

"Okay. Come get us then," he told me. "Or we can just go to the house tonight and meet you there when you get home."

That idea was a no-brainer and I knew Ed and I didn't even need to discuss it. We didn't trust Heather at our house with us away.

"No," I said. "We get in late tomorrow night and I need sleep. I will be there to pick you up first thing Monday morning."

Monday morning the sky was gray and the air was hot and humid, and I wondered if that was foreshadowing. I called my Research Assistant at George Washington University to let her know I was back from the conference but would not be at work that day. My insides were tight and shaking, bracing for unpleasant conflict, as I drove from our home in Silver Spring about fifteen miles out to the community of Gaithersburg where I parked the car and paused for a moment before I knocked on the apartment door. I had no idea what to expect. I only knew bits and pieces of the story.

Jeff and Heather, who had recently been evicted from the duplex they lived in next to Heather's mother and sister in western Maryland, were temporarily staying with friends. I knew these friends; they had been at my house numerous times. And I did not like them. Johnny and Amy had serious problems and he was a convicted, unregistered sex offender. I did not want him around my granddaughter Hannah and I had told Jeff and Heather that.

When Heather first told us that Johnny had been in prison for molesting his own daughter, whom he was no longer allowed to see, I said they should keep Hannah away from him.

"Oh, he wouldn't do anything to Hannah," she said with a giggle.

"Even if there is the remotest possibility that he might, you just can't have her around him," I said. Jeff agreed and told Heather I was right, but I kept seeing Amy and Johnny with them and Hannah when they visited us and I worried. I knew Heather always did whatever was easiest for her and not what was best for her child or anyone else. It was one of the reasons I did not trust her.

Jeff opened the door and stood back to let me into the apartment, and I took in the dismal scene in front of me. Heather sat slouched on the beat-up old sofa, staring straight ahead and paying no attention to her child or husband, and she ignored me as if she wished I would just go away, which I'm sure she did. She was sitting with Amy and Johnny while Jeff paced behind them gathering up suitcases.

Seated in a tired little lump on the floor, next to an old coffee table, her shoulders hunched and her eyes drooping as if she might fall over at any moment, was the newest love of my life. She looked at me in surprised recognition and held her thin little arms up. I went straight to her. She was the reason I was here. I was here to rescue Hannah, and I would help Jeff with whatever he needed to keep them both safe.

Hannah weighed only fifteen pounds and was as light as a feather when I pulled her up into my arms, and she smelled of wet diaper and dirty hair. My guess was she had not had a bath in at least a week and she looked exhausted so I knew she had not had enough sleep.

She greeted me with the sweet open mouth kiss of a baby, and then put her head on my shoulder and clung to me as if saying "please take me out of here." I hugged her tightly and headed for the door.

Jeff quietly picked up the two suitcases, walked with me toward the door, and said in a low voice, "Let's go."

"Isn't she coming with us?" I whispered, nodding in the direction of the sofa.

He shook his head, looking grim and determined as he marched forward, saying nothing to the people behind us. I followed him out in silence, holding Hannah close to my heart, and feeling a deep sense of relief when we were outside.

I was a little confused, afraid to believe this was what I hoped it was. Was he really leaving her at last? When we talked on the phone the day before, the plan was still that Jeff, Heather, and Hannah were all going to stay with us for an undetermined period of time.

As Jeff put the suitcases in the trunk of my Honda Accord, I stood on the sidewalk and gave Hannah a reassuring smile. "I promise I will never let you go back," I told her with tears in my eyes. She hugged me and put her head back on my shoulder, and I felt her sigh and knew that she understood I was making a commitment to her and that she was safe now. Jeff buckled her into the car seat I bought for her last year, and she quickly fell asleep as we drove away.

Later Ed and I talked in our room about what this meant for the future, and we were in complete agreement that Hannah's welfare was our primary concern. What a relief; at least we were not fighting like we did the year Jeff and Heather were first married. We'd been happy together for thirteen years and that was the only year we argued like that. Her behaviors and Jeff's attempts to defend her caused so much trouble in our house that it was like walking through a landmine all the time, and I was just glad we were now back to being happy together. I did not want that to change. But I was also determined to take care of Hannah and hoped he was too.

"This might be permanent," I warned him.

"I know that," he said, but I wondered if he really did, and if he had any idea what that would mean for us as a couple.

"Ed, you never raised a child, so I just wonder if you understand what you're getting into," I said. "You know?"

He looked at me, thinking for a moment before he spoke. I liked his hesitancy because it told me he was taking this decision seriously so I waited for him to respond. Sometimes my husband acts and speaks impulsively and with the sweet naiveté of a man who kept his life very simple until he met me.

"Look, I have already changed more diapers than Heather has," he said. "We are going to take care of that baby. That's all there is to it."

Ed is a man of commitment and when he says he will do something I know he will do his very best, so I believed him. "We will do whatever it takes to keep Hannah safe," he said.

I also knew that Ed wanted, maybe even more than me, to help Jeff get out of this crazy marriage. I didn't think we were always so angry at Heather, but her self-involved and abusive behavior toward Jeff and Hannah convinced us that she was not a very nice person and we didn't trust her with these people we loved so much. Lying in bed that night, with Jeff and Hannah safely sleeping down the hall from us, I thought back to how this all began. I couldn't help but wonder: could I have seen this coming and intervened? Of course then we wouldn't have Hannah and I would never have wanted that. Ed says Hannah is the reason it all happened and maybe he's right.

My love for Jeff has never wavered, but life with him has not been easy since his TBI in 1989. His choices, especially with women, have not been the best and it seems he has not learned from his mistakes like I knew he would have if he had matured into adulthood normally without injuring his brain. I think he would eventually have figured out what we all have to learn about who to trust and who not to trust.

When Jeff first called me, and I saw that there was a crack in his denial about Heather, I began to hope that the nightmare was going to end and that he would get out of the marriage.

It was an ordinary Friday morning and I was stuck in traffic on Route One, heading south from DC into northern Virginia, on my way to observe one of my graduate students doing an internship. Then my cell phone rang and everything changed.

"Hi. It's Jeff," he said.

"Yes, I recognize your voice." But he didn't laugh as he usually would.

"Well I have a question for you. What do you think is going on with Heather and Barney?"

This was a loaded question and I thought quickly before answering. Barney was a friend of Jeff's, someone he had known for years before either of them met Heather, someone we thought of as a "nice guy" who we were happy to have Jeff be friends with. Unlike some of his other friends who we were not so happy to have him hang out with, Barney was stable and he even had a job. But then Heather came along and Barney was not such a good friend to Jeff after all.

There were all of those phone calls Barney made to Heather, not Jeff, while they were visiting us. Then he would come to our house and he and Heather would giggle and talk privately. I had even watched them flirting and playing footsie at my kitchen table as if I was not standing right there.

"Jeff, are you okay with them going out?" I asked him one day when Heather went somewhere with Barney and left him at the house with us and the baby.

"They're just friends," he said.

I didn't think so and had been wrestling with whether to say something more to him. From prior experience with Jeff, Ed and I both worried about how he would react if I told him what I was seeing with her and other guys. I didn't want him to accuse me of trying to control his life.

Now he was asking me directly and I decided I should give him my honest opinion.

"I think they're having an affair," I said. "But what do you think?"

"I think so, too."

He began to tell me shocking stories like the night Barney drove all of the way from Montgomery County to western Maryland to pick Heather up for a party, leaving Jeff home alone with a sick baby who he said had a temperature of one hundred four degrees. He also had a fever and strep throat at the time, and that was the night he realized something wasn't right.

I was grateful that he was seeing reality but it made me sad that Jeff let this go on so long because I thought someone without a brain injury would have added it up long before that. Maybe not though; denial about spouses cheating is a universal problem for most of us.

"Tell me what you want and I'll do whatever you need to help," I said to calm him down.

"I want to leave and if I do Hannah comes with me."

My heart skipped a beat. I grinned from ear to ear there alone in my car, trying to pay attention to the traffic, and it was all I could do not to break out in a happy dance right there on the highway.

"Of course she does," I told him. "I can drive there and pick you up, just say the word."

"Thanks, I'll let you know," he said.

After I hung up with Jeff, I called Ed on my cell to tell him the good news that Jeff was coming to his senses, and then I went on to do my observation. My student was in crisis, having involved herself in a power struggle with her supervisor, and I had to focus on helping her to see her part in the problem. This student and I worked out a plan that made sense to both her and the supervisor who wanted to fire her from her internship. By the time I left I was tired and there was a lot of traffic so I got home late.

Over dinner Ed and I talked about how excited we were that Jeff was thinking of leaving Heather, but we both knew it might not happen. We had been down this road before and knew there were a lot of detours and pot holes to come; he could change his mind at any time and we had to tread carefully when we talked to him. He had to figure it out for himself, but oh-my-god it was hard to wait. It had been almost three years since they eloped.

"Remember?" Ed said. Of course I did. I'll never forget that day he told us he was married just like I will never forget February 17, 1989. Some memories are forever. But life goes on and we just had to adjust our sails in whatever storm we found ourselves boating through.

I was on an adrenaline rush now, in full rescue mode, determined to save Hannah from the bad life I believed she would have otherwise. Jeff needed our help with Hannah and the good news was that he knew it and admitted it. There had been a lot of times in the fourteen years since his car crash that it was like banging my head against a wall trying to get through to him, but like so many young people he had to learn from his own mistakes. The difference was that he repeated the same mistakes over and over, and some of the situations that he got into were really bad. He couldn't figure out what to do with the pieces after they all came crumbling down around him.

I loved my son but he was not the same as he was prior to February 17, 1989 and I was still getting to know the new Jeff. What happened to the old Jeff that day propelled our entire family onto a never before traveled road that we certainly would not have chosen if we had seen what lay ahead. I would have certainly selected a different future for myself and my kids if I could have.

ON JUNE 19, 2003 I wrote in my journal:

> *Things have changed so much in the past few months. The week before Easter Jeff and Hannah moved in here although I think at the time Jeff wasn't sure what he wanted to do. And now he has temporary custody of Hannah who is just so wonderful. Getting to help raise her is a thrill but so much work. I got very behind at GW last month but am slowly catching up.*

So Jeff moved in with us again, this time with a young lady we completely approved of and loved. I would do anything to keep Hannah safe and to help Jeff be the best father he could be because I knew how much he loved that little girl of his.

After Jeff and Hannah moved in with us, life became complete chaos again. Jeff was confused and depressed, and angry like all people are going through a separation. And Hannah was a baby who needed calm reassurance and protection as well as attending to her basic needs. I sometimes took Hannah to work with me to ensure her safety, and my students adjusted to me changing diapers while advising them or seeing me holding a baby in the back of the classroom while they did presentations.

One night as a student did her presentation for a class she stopped mid-sentence.

"Dr. Ruoff, I'm sorry but it's so strange to see you back there with a baby," she said. I held a sleeping Hannah in one arm and was taking notes with the other hand. I was getting used to it but realized it was incongruous for my students. We all laughed.

"I know. Just go on," I told her.

In my classes I made no secret about Jeff's brain injury and our complicated life, or our family issues, because I saw it as a valuable learning opportunity for them as education and human service professionals. There is so much more to the effects of brain injury than anyone can learn from reading articles, doing research projects, or learning facts. I wanted them to understand that a brain injury is not just a medical occurrence, but usually results in a life changing disability that affects the entire family for years to come.

"Jeff, do you mind if I talk about you when I'm teaching or doing presentations at conferences?" I asked him once.

"Nope. If it will help someone, go ahead and say whatever you want to," he said. Because Jeff was okay with it, I have always felt good that we are in agreement that we can tell our story openly. It's another way that I have let go of the secrecy and no-talk rules

I was raised with. And Jeff has said it makes him feel good if his experiences can help to educate others about TBI.

I know personally from my own divorce that the process is always hell for the people going through it, but for someone who has a disability like Jeff it becomes an extended family nightmare. The entire family went through Jeff's divorce with him. Ed and I went to every meeting with the attorney, every court hearing, and were involved with every decision.

Even though the initial decision to end his marriage was entirely Jeff's, I had to be involved every step of the way to protect Hannah and help him to get through it because of Jeff's severe memory deficits and confusion. After that first night in June, 2003, when I picked Jeff and Hannah up at Johnny and Amy's apartment, I called a lawyer I knew. She was part of a group of legal advocates for students with disabilities who were not being served appropriately by the special education system of the District of Columbia public schools and I had done some consulting with them as an expert witness on a few of their cases.

"Maggie, this is Janis Ruoff," I said. "I need some advice."

I explained the situation and said I thought we needed a good attorney who practiced family law and also understood disabilities. She gave me her recommendation and I called him. When he heard the short version of the story he said this kind of thing, in his experience, could turn into a crisis fast. So we set up an appointment for the next day and he gave me his cell number in case something happened. What great instincts that guy had; I liked him. He was nothing like my own divorce attorney which was a relief.

That night was a beautiful moonlit DC night, the last night of the first class for the summer session, and I gave my students a break before we did some wrap-up discussions. I walked outside the building and stood on the steps to get better reception and check my cell phone. There was a message from Jeff.

"May Day, May Day!" his voice said. "Call me please! This is urgent!"

I called and found out that Heather's mother was in our front yard with the police saying that we had kidnapped Heather and Hannah.

"Don't let her in the house," I told him. "I'll call you right back."

I found the cell number of the attorney, and when he heard what was going on he got our home number and called Jeff. He told Jeff to put the police on the line with him, and whatever he said to them caused them to leave and take Heather's mother with them.

I dismissed class early and ran to the opposite side of campus to find Ed who had begun taking graduate courses at GW toward a Master's degree. Looking through the window of the classroom door, I saw him standing in the front of the room doing his final presentation. He looked up to see me waving at him.

He came to see what was going on and when I told him he talked to his instructor, who let him leave. We then ran to the parking garage a few blocks away, found the car, and drove as fast as we could through Rock Creek Parkway to our house in Silver Spring. I was just glad it was after rush hour traffic and that Ed knew all the shortcuts; we got home in record time. I called Jeff to tell him we were on the way and he said the police had made Heather's mother leave.

When we walked into the house, not knowing what was going on, we found Jeff, Heather, and little Hannah all huddled together on our living room sofa. Heather said she told the police she did not want to leave with her mother and that she wanted to stay and work things out with Jeff. I was suspicious of her motives but we said we would support them in whatever they wanted to do.

When I called the attorney to tell him he said, "I want to see all of you in my office at ten in the morning," giving me the address.

The next day, Ed and I drove with Jeff, Heather, and Hannah to the office in DC and had a talk about what Jeff and Heather wanted to do. The lawyer told Heather about a job opportunity with a client of his, and made it clear he could not represent her if she and Jeff did get divorced. He would be Jeff's attorney at that point. Ed and I were impressed with him; he was smart and seemed to really know what he was doing and how to relate to everyone.

After a few days of uncertainty, Jeff's initial plans to work on the marriage were discarded when he took Heather to see her friends and heard Amy say, "Oh Heather! Barney called and said he still loves you and he bought you a ring!" I was home with Hannah when Jeff called me and said to pick him up, that he was done with Heather. It took two years and too many court hearings but Jeff and Heather were finally divorced, and Jeff got custody. We had the standard arrangement of visitation with Heather on weekends, and problems began right away because Heather could not manage having Hannah with her overnight.

A typical visitation weekend started with us driving almost an hour to take Hannah to Heather and Barney's apartment. A few hours later, about midnight, Heather would call to say Hannah wouldn't stop crying and wanted to come home. So Ed, Jeff, and I would get in the car and drive another hour and a half to get her and bring her home.

After those visits Hannah was anxious and clingy with me and cried easily. I would put her to bed in her room but she would always come toddling down the hall to climb into bed with us and would wrap her arms around my neck and sleep almost on top of me. Ed and I laughed because I got the hugs, kisses, and sweetness and she would put her bottom in Ed's face. He said he didn't mind though; he loved her no matter which end he got.

We quickly became a family of three parents and a toddler. Jeff found a job with Toys R Us close to our house and we juggled our schedules so that someone was always home with Hannah and she never had to have a babysitter. Every week we did a master family calendar that I posted on the kitchen wall. It enabled us to keep track of our busy lives and who was going to be home with Hannah or take her to preschool when she was old enough. It worked, and except for the tension around Jeff and Heather's divorce and ongoing legal battles we were all pretty happy.

Here I was in my fifties with a young child again, but my schedule at least was flexible and there were three adults in the house. Because of the wonderful research assistants I had, and the nature of a university, I could show up at my office late morning or early afternoon unless I had a meeting on campus, and that allowed me to drive Hannah to her preschool and make sure she had her lunch and whatever she needed for the day. Our morning routine became an important part of the day for both of us. I taught my classes in the evenings and by that time Jeff or Ed was there with Hannah and could pick her up if I wasn't available.

Hannah put on weight and began to thrive and grow after she was with us, and I saw her became a loving, cheerful, observant, and active little girl with a vivid imagination. She was so much fun to have around that it made up for any hardship.

"Let's play!" she would say the minute she got up in the morning. It was always important that I get up and have my first cup of coffee before I got her up because she popped out of bed wide awake.

"Okay. You're a kitty cat and I'm a monkey," I said one time. "And we are trying to stop Hannah from being such a good girl!" She loved that game. We called it the Mean Monkey and Mean Siamese Cat. I think the Siamese part came about because of the "We Are Siamese" cats' song from Lady and the Tramp.

"Yuck! Hannah's too nice!" I would say, which always set her off into giggles. "Let's do something diabolical and get her into trouble!" She would do whatever I wanted her to do just to hear that Mean Monkey frustrated, so that game and others like it kept her on track with getting dressed, eating breakfast, brushing her teeth, and all of the things she needed to do. A child's imagination is a wondrous thing and I loved every minute of sharing it with her.

When Hannah was a baby, still living with Jeff and Heather in western Maryland, we all settled on names for her to call Ed and me. When she tried to say Grandma and Grandpa I was Mamaw and Ed was Papa. Ed remained Papa, but after she was living with us she began to call me Mommy.

I was getting her ready for bed one night when she was about three years old and saw her looking sad. "What's wrong?" I asked. I felt her forehead, worried that she was not feeling well.

She looked at me thoughtfully and her response surprised me. "Would you be my mommy?" Her little face studied me and I saw this was a serious and important question to her and one I needed to respond to right away. But what should I say?

The problem was that I didn't know what to say because I didn't want to overstep my role, and I worried there could be legal complications if Heather heard her call me that. But I also knew how important it was for her to have someone in her life that she thought of as her mommy. I had asked my friends who were psychologists about it when Hannah first began calling me Mommy and they all said not to correct her.

"She's at risk for attachment disorder," one of them said. I looked that up on the Internet and as I read the reasons for, and ramifications of attachment disorder for children I realized how important this was for her to feel that security and attachment with me that she never felt with Heather.

Hearing her say out loud she wanted me to be her mommy, my heart melted into a puddle of mush. I put her on my lap and hugged her.

"You want me to be your mommy?" I asked her. She nodded still watching my face intently.

"Of course! You can call me anything you want to," I said. "But you do know I'm your grandma don't you?"

She nodded again and wrapped her arms around my neck.

"I already feel like your mommy anyway," I said. "So I can be

Mamaw and Mommy and, hey, now you have two mommies!" That made her smile and she seemed to relax. After that she always called me Mommy and later it became Mom. She also called Heather Mommy when she was with her, but I was the one raising her and taking care of her on a daily basis. And to a child, that's a mommy.

There is a lot to consider and sort out for families when grandparents and a biological adult parent are raising children together, and I've now met a number of "Grand Families" who struggle with a lot of challenges, some similar to ours and some very different. There are all kinds of reasons for whatever the arrangement is; in our case it was because of Jeff's disability and the fact that Hannah's mother did not and should not have custody.

Ed and I have often discussed that we cannot completely save Hannah from the life she was born to have, but we could do our very best to give her all the love and security possible and to help Jeff be the best dad he could be. Hannah understands it now and is wise beyond her years in the same way that many children raised in families like ours seem to be.

Jeff's TBI-related problems have presented unique challenges in what to say to Hannah and what not to say, and when to say it depending on her age and what she needed to know. Even though we always talked openly at home about Jeff's brain injury, there were a lot of things we never told Hannah because it would not be appropriate for her to know. Like the ongoing issues that came up because of Jeff's poor judgment, memory problems, and emotional ups and downs. Sometimes he was supposed to take her someplace and got the information all wrong and they ended up in the wrong place. Most of the time we could laugh off those confusions, but there were other situations that required more thought and problem-solving discussions among the three of us.

When Hannah was four years old she was out with Jeff one evening and I was home fixing dinner, when he called me on his cell phone.

"I need you to come get Hannah," he said. "I'm being arrested."

Fortunately he was only a mile from our house, so I drove to the location he gave me and found the police with Jeff on the side of the road. Hannah was sitting in the backseat, in her booster seat, all excited because Daddy was talking to the police. I talked to the police officer for a minute and learned Jeff had been stopped because, once again, he had speeding tickets and had not paid the fines so there was a bench warrant out for him that I had not known about.

I was furious with Jeff and yet had to act calm and smile so Hannah wouldn't worry.

"Daddy needs to help the policeman with something, so I'm taking you home," I said. "He'll be back later."

I told Jeff that one of us would meet him at the police station, and I switched Hannah to my car and got her out of there before he was handcuffed and taken away in a patrol car. She didn't need to see that.

When we got back to our house, I fed Hannah and got her ready for bed, trying to keep everything as normal as possible so she didn't worry. Ed picked Jeff up at the police station and they went back to get the car he was driving earlier that was still parked alongside the road on University Boulevard.

The police let Jeff go but he had to appear in court the next day and pay the fines he owed, and of course he did not have the money. We loaned it to him and then we all talked once again about the dangers of him speeding and that it was not acceptable for him to lie about the tickets he had received. He was embarrassed and remorseful, which was an improvement over previous times, but he seemed confused about why he did any of the things he was doing.

"Jeff, why would you speed after what happened to you?" I asked. "And Hannah was with you!"

I was convinced now that this was a reoccurring pattern; I was not imagining it and it wasn't just the effects of his TBI. Jeff's behavior was looking to me like a mania and depression cycle and not just the cognitive problems or depression so many people had from having a TBI and difficulty adjusting. He went into those long periods of depression, sleeping too much and watching TV, and then there were manic-like states of suddenly disappearing to have trysts with women he barely knew, or getting speeding tickets, starting a business he couldn't possibly do, and spending money on things he could not afford and did not need.

"Do you think he's bipolar?" I asked his neuropsychologist. "He has mood swings, and there are times when he can keep up with things and then suddenly he just can't."

"No, a TBI sometimes looks like bipolar disorder," he said. But I still had my questions and doubts. I began reading up on the dual diagnosis of TBI and mental health problems like bipolar disorder, and the more I read the more I became convinced Jeff had both. I felt he should have a dual diagnosis of TBI and Bipolar Disorder (BPD). I dropped it as life went on, but it remained a question in my mind that I thought about over and over, watching for further signs that I might be right about the BPD.

Jeff's job with Toys R Us ended because the company closed the store where he worked, and then he tried working for Starbucks. One complication with that job was that Jeff was a nice looking young single guy so many young, attractive women came into the store and wrote their phone numbers on napkins for him.

"It's like an alcoholic working at a bar," I told Jeff when he explained to me how distracting it all was for him.

"I know," he said with a grin. At least he was talking about it this time. He said he thought he was going to be fired anyway, but when I suggested we find a job coach he did not want that.

He was not fired for flirting with customers but because his supervisor said he didn't set up a display fast enough for her, which I thought was disability discrimination. I called the national office of the company and they said they did not discriminate so if there was such a problem I could call back. I was ready to help Jeff fight for his rights and stay on that job, but he said no, he thought he needed to move on to something else. He was probably using better judgment than me in that situation.

After Starbucks, Jeff went through a few sales jobs until he finally got a part-time job with the school district as a paraeducator. It provided a low-paying but steady income with good benefits, and he liked it. He had at one time wanted to be a teacher after all. Now he thought he was.

When people asked him what he did, he would say with pride," I am a teacher."

I was glad he had something he enjoyed and that he was willing to get up and go to work for every day. But, true to his pattern and history, he became romantically involved with one of the young teachers and over the summer was transferred to another school.

"Jeff, you have a problem with women, don't you?" I asked him. Sometimes I'm a little slow on the uptake when it's a person I love. I guess I didn't realize how much insight he had and I was surprised when he just laughed at me.

"Ya think?" he said, vowing to stay out of relationships at work.

The new school where Jeff now worked was close to our house and he could even walk there in good weather, so it felt like we were getting to a new era of stability. Ed finished his Master's degree and took a job with Special Olympics International that he was excited about. Hannah was getting older and her life was all about her Montessori school, piano and karate lessons, birthday parties, play dates on the weekends, and her visitation times with Heather which was now court-ordered to be supervised by us. On Sunday afternoons we met at McDonalds for two hours and Hannah played games with Heather, her mother, Hannah's aunt, Barney, and Hannah's two younger half-sisters while Jeff, Ed, and I sat in a booth nearby playing cards. To Hannah it was a big party and she loved it. For us, it was an improvement over the previous arrangements because at least we knew Hannah was safe, and that was the most important thing to us so we made the best of it.

Work was becoming complicated for me though. I had three federal grants, about a hundred students to advise and teach, and management of the Master's degree program and my graduate certificate program. I had contracts with state governments, the Veteran's Administration (VA), and other organizations to consult or teach classes for them. I taught both on campus and online classes and my involvement on boards and as a speaker at professional conferences was an ever increasing challenge that felt impossible at times. I was working all the time, even on weekends and evenings, whether it was professionally or taking care of Hannah. It was what I had dreamt of and I loved it, but I was beginning to wonder how long I could keep this up.

Because of the events of September 11, 2001 the military became interested in the problems of people with TBI and I was asked to help develop a film on TBI for the Army. Then I was asked to meet with high-level people at the Pentagon as they began to address the problems of returning soldiers who had sustained traumatic brain injuries from the roadside improvised explosive devices (IEDs). As I sat in a breakfast meeting one morning with the Acting Secretary of the Army and two other generals, talking to reporters with major newspapers, I wondered how the hell I got there. Me, the disgruntled Army wife and struggling doctoral student; there I was with this elite group talking about ways the Army could do better to help people with TBI and PTSD?

After that meeting I was contacted by a reporter for USA Today doing an article on the military and brain injuries; I was quoted on page one saying that if the military did not improve things it would all be up to the families. I felt like my work was making a real contribution to society and I was excited about the future and still had big plans for doing even more. This was the payoff; it was my time to do the things I had wanted to do when I worked so hard to finish my Ph.D.. And best of all Jeff seemed to be stable. He had been working for the school district for almost three years unless you counted the summers when he was not employed but did have ongoing benefits.

Then one morning, as Jeff was leaving for work I looked at him and saw it. I was learning to see and confront a lie instead of pretending it wasn't there. Something had changed with me. I knew Jeff was lying and something told me he no longer had a job.

"Jeff, you aren't going to work are you?" I asked him.

His mouth kind of fell open and he stared at me in surprise. I could almost read his mind: how the fuck did she know? He opened and closed his mouth a few times before he spoke.

"No. I quit," he said with his tilted head look of defiance.

Okay, so what was the story this time? It turned out to be familiar. Same old lie, different day and situation. He had been pretending to go to work for a whole month. Unbeknownst to me, or anyone else, Jeff had panicked because the principal put him on probation. There were complaints from a parent because he did not do something right and he thought he would be fired, so he just quit the job instead of trying to improve or get help. He went to the nearby shopping mall every day to just hang out and read until the time he would normally come home.

"Why would you do that?" I asked. "Why didn't you tell us you needed help?"

I was observing myself as if from a distance, thinking this was really stupid. I needed to stop asking Jeff these why questions because he never knew the answers and it didn't matter anyway. For the first time since his TBI I saw that maybe I was holding him to a standard of normalcy that he could not reach and that my expectations were too high. But I was angry at him, at the principal of the school for putting him in that position, and at myself for once again being duped by a lie and too busy to see the signs that Jeff needed help. Was it too late? Could I rescue him for this one last time? It was such a good job for him and I wanted to make this all go away.

I gave it my best effort. We went to the school and talked to the principal but it was too late to change anything and reinstate him. His lies had let too much time pass before I knew and was able to intervene on his behalf.

"I was surprised when he quit and tried to talk him out of it," the Principal said and I understood his perspective. Jeff had the right to quit his job and he was an adult so for his boss to call his mom would be illegal and disrespectful. I would have done the same thing, although probably I would have suggested he see someone in the Human Resources office for help. Principals are busy though and they don't always understand disabilities even for their own students much less the staff.

With Jeff once again unemployed, and the rest of us still on the busy Washington DC treadmill, Jeff was alone at the house during the day. He went into a depression again, not getting up in the morning and sleeping off and on all day. I was too busy to deal with it though, and it was all I could do to take care of Hannah and keep up with my work. I just wanted Jeff to stay home to rest and minimize the chaos while we tried to figure this out.

"Don't look for any other jobs, okay?" I said when Ed and Jeff and I discussed what had happened. "We all need time to think about this."

A few weeks later Ed and I were asleep when the phone next to our bed rang and woke me up. It was Jeff and at first I was disoriented because I thought he was in his room sleeping.

"Where are you?" I asked.

"I'm leaving," he said. "I just called to say goodbye and thank you for everything."

Was he serious? I looked over at Ed who was awake now, watching and waiting. My stomach lurched and tears began to cloud my vision.

"It's Jeff," I whispered to Ed. "He's not in his room."

"Jeff, where are you? We'll come get you. I love you and it will all be okay. Don't move, just sit down and wait!"

He began to cry and told me he was on a street corner on Connecticut

Avenue, in DC, and he agreed to wait. I stayed home with Hannah who was asleep in her room, and Ed went to pick Jeff up.

When they got home I hugged my tall, grown up but very confused son and we sat down to talk.

"Jeff, we all love you, and Hannah needs you. You can't do this."

"That's why I called," he said. He explained that he felt useless, and that he planned to just keep walking until he dropped and died. It made no sense to me but it did to him, and that was the problem.

The next day I took him to a local hospital that I knew had a good psychiatric inpatient program. He was admitted voluntarily for evaluation and stayed there a week, during which time he was diagnosed with bipolar disorder (BPD) by the resident psychiatrist. They started him on mood stabilizing medication and he attended intensive group therapy. When they discharged him it was with medical orders for ongoing treatment through their all-day outpatient mental health program, and a follow-up visit with the consulting psychiatrist.

I was so relieved because this was the missing part to the big picture, and explained so much about why Jeff could not maintain employment and stability no matter how hard he tried or how much support we all gave him. I decided that our life was just too complicated for any of us to manage. Sometimes I have to keep crashing into those walls over and over before I decide to make whatever changes are needed. But this did it for me.

"We need to simplify," I said to Ed. "Jeff can't keep up with the pace of life here in Montgomery County, and I am afraid I can't continue doing what I'm doing."

We began talking seriously about moving, but there was so much to consider: my work at GW, Ed's job, the Montessori school Hannah and we were all involved with, and friends we had known for a lifetime. Then there was the issue of taking Hannah somewhere else and how Heather would react. It was a hard decision and we continued to talk but couldn't see a clear path.

There were too many choices and options and we did not know what would work out the best.

In the November of 2009 Hannah turned eight and one night not long after that I came home from a long day at work, having spent all day in tedious faculty meetings and budget discussions, then teaching an evening class. I wasn't home in time to say goodnight to Hannah but she was awake waiting for me, and heard me come in, so I went to her room to hug and kiss her and tell her I would drive her to school in the morning. She smiled and went to sleep.

I said goodnight to Jeff who was reading a book in his room across the hall from Hannah, and went to our bedroom to get undressed and talk to Ed.

"How is my favorite person in the whole wide world?" he asked me. I burst into tears.

"I'm exhausted! I just can't do this," I told him. "It's too much and they're pushing me to write another grant and bring in more money. And when I did spread sheets for the budget it just doesn't work; another grant will give me more work than I can manage and won't allow me to hire help and pay my salary at the same time, so I can't do it. I'm so tired and frustrated!" I was sobbing by then.

"What do you want?" he asked. "Is there something I can do?"

I knew that it was up to me to decide what I needed and then Ed would help me. I was married to a very different man now than I was years ago. I always jokingly told Ed, "You are the best husband I ever had," but I meant it. Ed was truly my partner and we could work this out. I'd been thinking about this for a long time and it was suddenly clear that night that the old feeling of being stuck in a box was back and I was keeping the walls in place like I used to do.

"It's our whole lifestyle," I said. "I need for us to change everything. We have to make some big changes, okay?"

I showed him the notes I had scribbled while riding the metro home that night. I had calculated how much of my time was spent on what I wanted to be doing and it was not much. What I was spending a lot of time doing, at least four or five hours every day, was driving in traffic or taking a crowded metro train back-and-forth.

"What can we do so you can be happy?" he asked me. "If you keep going I'm afraid you'll have a nervous breakdown." I started to argue but realized he might be right. I no longer wanted to be a superhero and do it all.

I read a book on making life changes and it said when there is confusion about what to do you need to do more research. I needed to find out information and so I made a list of my research questions. Should I leave GW? How could we make this work financially? If we moved, and I wasn't sure we had to, where would we go? Ed and I decided the first thing to do was to find out if and when I could retire from my job instead of just quitting. I did not want to leave my mission of teaching about brain injury behind and I had always planned to work, doing whatever I was doing, until I was so old I couldn't, but that was before Jeff's TBI and before Hannah.

I set up an appointment with a woman who handled retirement for faculty at GW and Ed went with me. We learned that I could take early retirement in January of 2011 if I wanted to and Ed looked at me with excitement.

"You should do it!" he said. "I can work and support us, and you can stay home with Hannah, help Jeff, write, and do what you want to do."

I was intrigued by the prospect of retiring and yet scared of the loss of my income after the years of living financially on the edge as I had when I first met Ed. I'm a social liberal, maybe even a little bit of a free spirit when I let myself be, but I'm also a financially cautious person and it seemed impossible to me that we could make this work if I was not earning money.

"If we don't have my salary we can't afford to stay in our own house living here, so we'll have to move," I said. "Do you really want to leave DC?" Ed had lived there all of his life and I had thought I would live in the DC area the rest of mine. I still loved so much about the east coast and the Washington DC communities.

He smiled. "Let's see. Our house was broken into this year by thieves while we were all sleeping, we have rats invading and setting up homestead inside our walls, Jeff can't keep a job here, and we are paying all of this money for private school, commuting, and high Montgomery County taxes. Hmmmm. Should we move? Yes, I want to move."

The second thing on my list of questions was: where could we live that we could afford if I stopped working? I didn't know. And there was another possibility to explore: could I continue working part-time and still maintain our lifestyle in the DC area? I was pretty sure the answer to that was no.

Planning our new future became our favorite topic and provided us with endless dinner conversations for our Friday night dates which Ed and I had made a regular part of our life. On Friday nights we went out alone so we could talk, and we gave Jeff money to order pizza for him and Hannah. Everyone loved it.

One Friday night Ed and I went to our favorite Outback restaurant, waited the usual forty-five minutes for a table, and got into decision making. There was so much to consider but we agreed it made sense to explore moving away to an entirely new area. In a year and a half Hannah would be finished with third grade, and if we were to move somewhere else that would be a good age for her before she got into middle school.

Ed and I began looking at options and took short trips to nearby states and locations further out in the DC suburbs of Maryland and Virginia. And I stopped writing grant proposals.

SECTION III

Alice: How long is forever?
White Rabbit: Sometimes, just one second.

—Lewis Carroll, Alice in Wonderland

A quote from Alice in Wonderland by Lewis Carol can apply to my life. The King states: "Rule 42. All persons more than a mile high have to leave the court." I apply this quote to myself because I spent about two decades in denial about being disabled. That is twenty years of having an over-inflated ego and ceaselessly entering relationships and jobs that I should not be in. Now I have right-sized myself and am living a much happier life.

—Jeff Bouck, TBI Survivor

Chapter 11

My New Script

SOMETIMES YOU JUST HAVE TO rewrite your own life story and decide how you as the protagonist want to see it turn out. Even though I know living in the moment is the key to happiness, planning a different path and moving in a new direction can lead to more of the kind of moments you want. This was a story about our family after Jeff's TBI and me who wanted a more stable and happy family life but could not find it for a long time. Now I have a new script for my life. I am no longer a woman who wants change; I don't fear change but now I want to keep my life as it is and that's something remarkable to me.

2016

I GET A TEXT SAYING "Mom! I'm hungry!" It's Hannah who is upstairs in her room; I'm in the kitchen below so why can't she just come down and get something to eat? She's fourteen and she's part of that generation, the ones who cannot imagine what life was like when there were no cell phones or iPods. I send a text back. "So... your point is?" I add emojis: smiley face, quizzical face, cool face with sunglasses.

She shows up then to get a snack and go back to her room for more texting with her friends. She's supposed to be doing homework but I know she isn't. She just likes being in her room where she imagines she has no parents, I presume. That is until she needs me to cook for her or take her to her Taekwondo classes, or when she misses the school bus. I've come full circle back to being the mom of a teenager again but with a lot of differences from the days when Jeff and Travis were this age. I'm much more present and involved.

I go back to fixing dinner: a huge salad, vegetables and beans or cheese for me because I'm vegetarian now, and I make extra vegetables for everyone else to have with their meat dishes. Dinner at our house is a little crazy with everyone eating different things, and sometimes being on different schedules, but life is good. We all eat healthy and we have the lifestyle I was hoping we would have when we moved to Colorado.

In January, 2011 I took early retirement from GW and we decided to move away from our life in Washington DC to somewhere, but we didn't know where. Jeff said he didn't care; he was just excited about starting a new life without the reminders of all of his past mistakes and failed relationships with women who all still called him on days like Valentine's Day or around the Christmas holidays. But it wasn't easy to make the decision.

"In more ways than one it's going to be hard to leave this place," I told my friend Betsy when we had lunch one day and I explained what we were thinking of doing. I knew I was going to miss her and all of the other friends we had known for so many years.

"Couldn't you just move somewhere close by?" she asked.

"We've looked at a lot of places near DC and it just doesn't work for us," I said. "Everywhere we looked it's too expensive, still too much traffic, and in some cases not good schools. Besides, we need a slower way of life."

Something in me was shifting. Was it because I was getting older, or was I just that tired out? My desire to change the world was beginning to fade and I was more interested in making the simple changes at home so that our family could manage life better. My mother, who died a few years after my father, loved slogans and her constant words of "charity begins at home" floated through my head like some spiritual guidance, reminding me that I had a lot of saving still to do with our family.

When we started the process of selecting a new place to move to I wrote out lists of what Ed and I each wanted, supports I thought Jeff needed and what I believed Hannah needed to grow up to be a healthy and happy young woman. Excellent schools and a safe community were at the top of my lists.

I sat at my computer searching for information on places we could relocate to that would give us what I knew we needed. I had my checklist: good schools for Hannah, a safe and friendly community that Jeff could navigate better, decent medical care and disability supports, a lower cost of living, plenty of activities we could all enjoy, and lots of sunshine because I decided maybe I have seasonal affective disorder. I was always depressed during the dark days of winter. I wanted a lower cost of living, lots of sunshine, friendly people, and a nice house we could afford with enough space for all of us so we weren't too cramped. Ed especially wanted a place with a strong sports community for his sports officiating, close proximity to an airport for travel, and good Internet so he could work from a distance. We both wanted more freedom, somewhere Hannah could go out to play without us worrying about her safety, and most of all no Norway rats or thieves crawling in the windows.

"Hey, I think I've found it!" I said to Ed. "I searched on two things: best places to retire and best places to raise a child."

I showed him what I found and there were only two cities that came up on both of my search results. One was the Raleigh Durham, North Carolina area and the other was a city we had never visited called Fort Collins in northern Colorado.

We had been to North Carolina many times exploring both the beach towns and the Raleigh Durham area, and we liked that option except that my allergies were terrible there. And when I mentioned to one of the research assistants in our office at GW that I was thinking we should relocate close to a beach he cautioned me against it. He grew up in one of the communities we were exploring.

"Too much partying there," he said. "You don't want to raise Hannah at the beach."

"I would love to live near the mountains!" Ed said. I saw the glow in his eyes and could read his mind; he was envisioning the great escape, the geographic cure. Move out west and be a free spirit, drive all over to different mountain towns, go hiking and fishing! Have fun, just like a vacation all of the time! He's an escape junkie.

"Hey, slow down," I said. "We are looking for a good place for normal life," I reminded him, sorry that I was deflating his enthusiasm but needing a realistic plan. The last thing I wanted was to do this and find that it didn't work out.

"Let's go see it," he said. I suspected he just wanted to go on another vacation out west, but I also knew it was important for both of us to experience a place, to get the feel of it, and to look at houses to see what we could afford.

"I know someone who lives in Fort Collins," I said, suddenly remembering a friend who had moved there. "I could call Kim and ask if we could visit them for a few days. She invited me last time she was here."

The Callahans are a couple with a son named Kit who had a TBI two years after Jeff's injury. Their family was active in brain injury support groups in Virginia. Kim and I served on the Board of Brain Injury Services in Virginia for years and had talked a lot about the challenges of having a young adult child with a TBI. When they moved to Colorado, Kit went with them so I knew she could also tell me about the resources she had found for Kit in that state and that would help us in making our decision. I also knew their daughter and son-in-law moved to Fort Collins not long after they did and they had a daughter Hannah's age. I thought it would be good to introduce the girls and they could tell me about the schools and activities for kids.

Every year we joined our friends in the Virginia brain injury community for the Kit Callahan Miracle Mile, a run that was a fundraiser for Brain Injury Services, and at the last one Kim had pictures of their new home. It looked beautiful.

"Great!"

Ed was off and running looking for bargain airfare before I even called Kim.

When I did call, her response was "Sure! We'd love to have you visit!"

The trip was just what we needed to make a decision; we would move to Colorado at the end of Hannah's third grade. That gave us a little over a year to get our house ready to sell, look for a new place in Fort Collins, and for me to begin backing off from boards and my commitments in the DC area.

"Ed, are you sure?" I asked him over and over.

"We need to use the Prayer of Increase Decrease," he said. "If we are meant to move to Colorado that path will increase, and if not it will decrease." It was like the God Box he told me to use in 1990. I wasn't comfortable with that approach, because it meant too much letting go of control, but decided once again to try it.

And things just began falling into place. We flew out to Fort Collins a second time and narrowed our house search to a few neighborhoods we liked, and finally found what we were looking for.

READY TO CROSS THE NEXT HURDLE, I called Heather to talk to her and work things out for maintaining communication and visits after we moved, and she agreed to have lunch with us. But when we drove to her apartment an hour away we discovered that she had left and after that she refused to talk to us. Instead she did what we expected and forced us back into court. I felt great sympathy for her because of course she did not want her daughter to move away. If I were her I would probably fight us too. But I knew—we all knew—that this was the best thing for Hannah and the judge agreed. We got legal permission to move Hannah to another state, and we also got the custody arrangement changed so that Jeff, Ed, and I have a three-way joint custody now.

The signs kept increasing for us to move, telling us we were heading in the right direction. We sold our house and put a contract on the new one. We would move as soon as school was out the second week of June.

Hannah was not completely convinced that moving was a good idea because she was a child and wanted to stay with her friends and what she knew. But she'd met the Callahans' granddaughter when we took Jeff and Hannah with us one time to visit Colorado, so she was aware that she would not be friendless in her new home and that helped. She was getting used to the idea of moving and accepting it. But as moving day grew closer Hannah became worried that we would give her toys away.

As a child growing up with doting grandparents and a father who would give her anything he could, Hannah had enough stuffed animals and toys to start her own toy store, and we all understood why it was important to take them all with us. She was leaving her mother and sisters and the only life she had ever known.

Those stuffed animals all had names and life stories, and they were a part of her family to her. Whenever a new one came to live with us I had to introduce it to all of the others and explain why he or she was there. "My name is Ralph the Bear and I used to live in a department store but my mommy was sold and Hannah saw me and bought me...." Or something like that.

"No toys left behind!" we all yelled as we tossed one toy after another into six large boxes for the move. We took turns speaking for the toys.

"Don't forget me! I want to go live in Colorado!" they each said. Hannah laughed and got caught up in the game, and that's how we got her to pack for the move. The Mean Monkey and Mean Siamese Cat even made an appearance and said they were going to follow us out west, to which Hannah and I both said, "Oh no!"

On a sunny day in mid-June, after an exhausting week of packing and cleaning, our friends picked us up to take us to the Reagan National Airport in DC. These friends were people we had become close to, sharing a common bond of pain and frustration, and love for our granddaughters, who were sisters. They were the parents of Heather's husband Barney. But that's another story so you will have to read my next book to find out more.

As we fastened our seat belts and got ready for take-off we gave each other a high-five.

"We did it!" I said.

Unlike the flight I remembered all too well on February 17, 1989, I could look over and see Jeff sitting right there across the aisle.

"How you doing?" I asked him. He gave me a thumbs up and grinned from ear to ear.

We have never regretted the move, and for me I know that becoming a full time mom for Hannah, case manager for Jeff, and exploring other pursuits like writing is what I was meant to do at this point in my life.

The time came, before we left for our new life in Colorado, when I knew Jeff could no longer sustain employment. "Jeff, it's time for you to get SSDI," I told him. "And this time I'm going to get us some help."

I talked to a colleague and friend, a lawyer specializing in TBI, and he helped me put together the information for reapplying for SSDI once we were settled in our new home. SSDI applications are all about getting the right story together and in most cases having a lawyer involved. We got an updated neuropsychological evaluation from a well-known neuropsychologist who said Jeff did well on paper tests, which made him look employable, but that he had "failed the test of life." That was hard to read but sadly I knew it was true, at least with employment and independence. It was twenty years of Jeff trying so hard to get and keep jobs and always finding himself out of work and depressed, and now there was the new diagnosis of BPD in addition to his TBI. This time I felt like it all made sense for Jeff to stop working and get the support he deserved. In the past I was reluctant to help him push for that because I wanted to believe he could be normal, whatever that is, and because I thought having the label of permanently disabled would take away his motivation. I suppose it all worked out how it was meant to be, but I feel a great deal of sympathy for people trying to get help.

We decided to wait to file a new claim in our new location so that we got to know the people with the local Social Security Offices. Jeff does receive SSDI now and he also has support through the county's mental health programs with regular therapy appointments and groups and new friends. Most importantly, he now stays out of destructive dating relationships. When we talk about his problems in the past with women, which he describes as a relationship addiction, I tell him it's kind of like me trying to avoid overeating and he says "Mom, a cheesecake doesn't pick up the phone and call you." He has a good point there and I admire him for letting go of the cheesecakes in his life. He's stable now and he doesn't lie to me anymore, or if he does it only lasts a few minutes and he apologizes. Then he forgets it happened so he repeats the same mistakes at another time. It's who he is and acceptance has taken many years but I think I'm there now.

Sometimes, once or twice a month, we drive to Denver, or we go to one of many mountain towns in our new home state. As we drive pretty much anywhere we see the mountains in the background and we always talk about what a beautiful place we live in and congratulate ourselves on this decision.

Our move has been good for Hannah. She's in wonderful schools and we live in a safe community, and she has become a beautiful and well-adjusted teenager who cares about people and has goals in life. She enjoys music and plays the piano, guitar, and violin. She is working to get her black belt in Taekwondo this year and she's a state champion in sparring and forms for her age group and rank. She's capable of taking care of herself when she needs to and she does things around the house when asked.

Every time I take Hannah back to the DC area for a visit I appreciate life in northern Colorado even more because the traffic gets worse every year back east. But I love catching up with the people who are still important to me. Fortunately, now we have cell phones and social media, and some of our old friends visit us now and then.

I often say, "If I wasn't me I'd be jealous of me." I have that life, that different life, I wanted back in 1989. We have busy times but they are not frenetic and we keep it as simple as possible. We still do a family calendar for the week so that we all remember who is taking Hannah to her lessons, picking her up from school, when Jeff has appointments, or who needs which car. But if someone forgets something it's not the big deal it was when life was so complicated.

One thing I love now is that if Jeff forgets something we can easily reschedule an appointment, and if I'm busy Ed or Jeff can go get Hannah at school if she misses the bus or pick her up when she's visiting a friend. With his TBI, and difficulties juggling priorities, I don't think I ever realized before how much Jeff needed this calmer life and simplicity until we finally had it. In this environment he functions so much better. People with brain injuries have reported that thinking after a TBI is like going from an automatic transmission in the car to a manual shift. And that's tiring. Jeff takes a lot of naps even now because of his mental fatigue, sleep problems, and side effects from medications, and our new lifestyle allows that.

What scares me as the mother of a teenager once again is that in less than two years Hannah will be old enough for her driver's license, and in just three years we will be helping her apply to colleges. I don't know how we are all going to let go of her but I know we will have to at some point. It will be hardest for Jeff I think because he's built so much of his life around being Hannah's dad, but I will help him to see what a good job he's done and how important it is to let her grow up.

In November of 2015 our dear friends, the Callahans, lost their son Kit. On a Tuesday morning I got an email from Kim saying he was in the hospital and I went to be with them before he died the next day, and then we all went to his funeral on Sunday and Monday. It's unclear whether the blood clots and other health problems Kit had were directly attributable to his TBI in 1992 but I think there is at least an indirect connection. Many people develop health problems related to either the diminished capacity to care for themselves after a TBI or to systemic problems that affect their brain and other parts of the endocrine or nervous system. None of that matters though. What matters is that after spending many years caring for and loving Kit back to having the best life he could have, as long as we have spent with Jeff, they have lost him at an early age and now they have to grieve all over again.

I talked to Kit's sister at the funeral and through her tears she looked at me and said, "Now what? All this time it's been all about Kit and now he's gone." I can only imagine how hard that would be and every time I get frustrated with Jeff, on the days when he has those out-of-it times that I call TBI moments, I remind myself that yes we are lucky as people said in 1989 when I hated them for saying it. We are lucky to still have him with us, no question, and I hope it goes on and on.

They say the only things we can really change in life are ourselves. I know I have changed and learned so much about living with someone who had a brain injury, and about family life and myself in the past twenty-six years.

Last year I almost got involved with the enormous and important topic of human trafficking but I decided but there are only so many things I can take on in this lifetime. If I could I'd like to stop all child abuse, human trafficking, animal cruelty, and murders. Maybe, if there is reincarnation, I'll get a chance to tackle some new things the next time around, who knows? But for now I focus on family needs and the smaller things that I feel I can make a difference with. For example, two years ago I decided to do something I wanted to do when I was a child. I wanted to get involved in raising a service dog for someone with a disability after I read a book called Follow My Leader by James Garfield (1957) when I was nine or ten years old. The book, which I still have on my bookshelf, is based on the author's life and is about a boy named Jimmy blinded by a firecracker during a Fourth of July accident and his seeing eye guide dog named Leader. I loved that book and read it over and over. I don't know why this story fascinated me except that I always loved animals and was drawn to people with disabilities. Also I was born with some vision problems, including amblyopia which Hannah inherited from me, so I grew up with an intense fear of becoming blind.

I searched the Internet and decided to apply to an organization called Canine Companions for Independence (CCI) to be one of their puppy raisers. After phone interviews, and a visit from someone who lived in our area and who had raised dogs for CCI, I was approved. I immediately called a family meeting.

"We are going to have to do this as a family," I said and everyone nodded. "That means we all have to study the Puppy Raiser manual together and agree on how to handle Buster when he gets here, right?"

"I'll do it!" Hannah said. She loves dogs.

As we read through the manual and discussed how to do housebreaking and teach commands, and that we would all need to be consistent, everyone got excited about it and it became a family commitment.

In June, 2014 Ed and I drove to the Denver airport and picked up an adorable mixed Labrador and Golden Retriever named Buster

IV. When I heard his name for the first time I told the CCI puppy coordinator, "He sounds like a CEO!" And he thought he was.

Buster was quite the noisy little guy, barking all the time, and very energetic. He hated his crate and for the first month barked so much that I began to think this might be a mistake. But as time went on he calmed down and I learned how to handle him, and our whole family became involved in this wonderful world of people and puppies for CCI.

Raising and training Buster was an unplanned part of our life but such a wonderful experience for all of us. Jeff took him to his therapy groups and out to meet with friends for hikes, and Ed and I took him on day trips and walks in the neighborhood. Hannah helped with his training and enjoyed the times he went with me to her school for back to school night, orchestra concerts, and to her piano recitals. He became a part of our life.

But the arrangement with CCI is that puppy raisers get a two-month-old puppy and keep him or her until the puppy is eighteen months old. So in November, 2015 Ed and I flew with Buster to turn him in for his advanced training at the facilities of CCI in Oceanside, California.

We were standing by the parking garage of the Santa Ana airport trying to find the rental car place with Buster on his leash by my side in a sit-stay position, when a voice next to me said, "Hey!"

I looked up and it was Travis! I had not seen him in a year because they live across the country from us and are very busy, and because Travis has been somewhat distant in recent years. I've missed him.

It was one of those moments that felt completely spiritual to me, and even more so later when I talked to him on the phone. He's now going through some midlife changes and has asked me to help with my grandson, and I'm happy I can be there for him the way he tried to be for me when he was a teenager. That chance encounter has led us back together.

Even if Buster does not make it all the way through his advanced training to be a service dog, and comes home to be a pet, he will have done a huge service for all of us. If not for him I would not have been in that spot on that day in California when Travis happened to be there on a business trip.

As I watched Buster leave us to go with his new trainer, looking back at me briefly as he was led to the kennel dormitory where he would live for six months with other CCI puppies, I felt grateful to have had the opportunity to make a difference in someone's life with that dog. His reports are good and we are planning that we will all go for his graduation soon to meet the person with a disability who he begins his life of service with.

Last month Hannah had spring break from school and we took everyone to Moab, Utah, which is a place Ed and I used to enjoy visiting before we were married. Moab is a funky town in the middle of red rock canyons and fascinating national parks with rock formations to climb and explore. We spent the week climbing, hiking, and just having a lot of fun. Hannah's part Billy goat and she was all over the place. The pictures I got of her standing on high rocks with her arms in the air and a gorgeous, colorful canyon behind her are priceless.

I wonder about something. There were those baby dreams that I had after my hysterectomy, dreams Dr. Stone and I disagreed about as to their meaning. And then there was the vision I had of a man sitting on the sofa and a child playing in front of him. Was that man Ed? Was that abandoned baby on the porch, the one crying and holding her arms out to me, a glimpse into the future? At that time I had no prospect of ever having a baby again, and I did not have a daughter like I do now. It gives me chills to think that I might have seen Hannah in that dream ten years before she was born. But maybe, just maybe I do have some sort of destiny after all.

Jeff and I have a tradition that we started back in Maryland many years ago. Every year we go out to lunch and see a movie together on February 17, which he calls his real birthday. We always talk about how far he's come and how great life is the second time around. And I always tell him how proud I am of him for his perseverance and his determination to get through all that he has.

When I have my seventieth birthday, which is not too far off in the future, I have decided I want to celebrate by climbing again to the top of Delicate Arch in Arches National Park. I want to look out over the canyon, feel the breeze and sunshine, and be healthy and strong enough to be fully alive and enjoy many more years of this great new life. I tell Hannah I plan to live another thirty years at least so I can follow her around and bug her.

I try not to think about the possible wreckage of the future anymore. I could of course, but Jeff with his TBI, Hannah with her optimism and enthusiasm for life, and Ed with his faith in a Higher Power have taught me to live one day at a time. And now I live with no walls, just the beautiful Rocky Mountains and wide open spaces of Colorado around me.

Chapter 12

If I Ruled the World

I SIT AT MY DESK WRITING THIS MEMOIR, and from the window I see a beautiful view of the Rocky Mountains which at this time of the year are snow-capped and majestic with the sun shining on them during the day and beautiful sunsets some evenings. We live in a place where people don't ask "What do you do for a living?" Instead someone would be more likely to ask, "Do you ski?" or "Where do you go hiking?" Our longest commutes to anything are usually ten minutes, twenty at the most, unless we are spending a few days in the mountains which we love to do when we can.

Life is so much easier to understand in the rear view mirror than it is when you are heading down whatever road you take and don't know where you are going. I have changed and so has Jeff, and from all that I have learned I feel like a much better driver now and I think he does too. It's not all about his TBI, but that one moment in time when he crashed into a van on the street we lived on in Maryland has been a catalyst for so much change in my life and for our entire family. I look back on it a lot, especially because I've been writing this memoir, and I see how well we all handled things even though it didn't seem like it at the time.

When I saw the signs telling me I needed a new script for my life, I didn't know how to write it or make it happen so I just turned it all over to that spiritual guidance I heard, a force of the universe, and asked for help. To my surprise it has worked so much better than when I had all of those goals posted on my bedroom wall, even though I think that was helpful at the time. I've made changes in all of my relationships so that I feel like they are now in the right place in the puzzle of my life.

I've learned so much about living with someone who had a brain injury, and about family life and myself in the past twenty-six years since I was pulled from that airplane on February 17, 1989. At that time of my life, living in fear, I was all about trying to plan and control the future but now I know I can't. I still have goals and dreams and hopes but I know that the changes that can occur are beyond my capacity to predict and I just need to accept them and adjust to whatever life brings.

Ed and I are aging but I don't like to admit that to myself, and we are still healthy and active. We have to be because we are parents of a teenager who still has so much life to live that we want to be a part of. Other couples our age might be able to completely retire and travel but that's not our life. And that has its positives and negatives like anything else.

I miss my university teaching at times, but I enjoy being Hannah's mom and writing, and Ed is happy doing more refereeing and some substitute teaching. Telecommuting was working fine for him after we first moved, and he planned to keep working until he got to be seventy or older, but last summer his job with Special Olympics was phased out. He was shocked and upset at first but as time goes by we see that it has been a good thing because he is enjoying life more. It's just one more reminder that life doesn't always go in the direction we plan, but maybe it's turning out however it's supposed to be. We are a family, a three generation family, and it works for us. For some other people it might not.

Every person is different, every family is different, and we bring all of our uniqueness to that horrible, dramatic moment when a child or adult suffers a TBI, aneurysm, stroke, gunshot wound, fall, or other event that damages the brain. In our case Jeff's car crash came at a time of transition for everyone in the family. He was finishing high school; I wrestled with multiple problems in my life; my ex-husband, Steve, was going through his own midlife crisis; and Travis was doing his best to cope with being a teenager in the midst of all of it. Obviously no one planned on something like that happening in our family, and we had no time to prepare. We just reacted. We were ordinary human beings when an extraordinary thing happened to us.

For some families, life changes early if a child who is young has a TBI and the parents, who may also be young, suddenly have to learn about rehabilitation and special education at the same time they're grieving over losing the child they had and all of their hopes for his or her future. Other families may develop a more gradual awareness that someone has been repeatedly injured from blows to the head during a favorite sport; they may need to see the results of neuropsychological and medical testing to understand that new, aberrant behaviors were caused by repeated concussions that created a brain injury. For some families their worst fears come true when a family member in the military is hurt by a roadside bomb that explodes near him or her. A brain injury can happen to anyone; it might be a person enjoying a much-needed vacation skiing who crashes into a tree or someone who goes out to get the mail after an ice storm and slips, falls, and hits the back of his or her head on the pavement. There are numerous causes of TBI and each person and each person's brain is different so affected in a unique manner.

Imagine this is happening to you. Regardless of how injury to the brain occurs, you—a mother, father, brother, aunt, wife, or best friend—gets a call saying that something has happened. At first it is a nightmare you can't wake up from. After some time it is just your life, but not the life you had expected and planned for. What would you do? I always liked something the people with the Brain Injury Association of Florida said: brain injury is the last thing on your mind until it's the only thing.

There are all kinds of families, but regardless of the special nature of a family's legal and emotional ties, whether people live together or apart or a mix of the two, a family is an interconnected system. The individual people in a family are all affected by each other's lives whether we like it or not. Even with a cut-off relationship like after a divorce or estrangement like I had with my parents, the connection of the mind and spirit remains. And family tragedy affects most of us like none other.

From my own experience, and what I have learned about families over the years, I can say with some degree of certainty that a brain injury sets up a new family life that is like Whack-A-Mole, the popular arcade game we play at the beach. Something unexpected pops up, you hit it down, and then another challenge pops up. Jeff decided to go away to college; I arranged it and thought I could focus on my dissertation; then he got involved with a con artist and had to quit school for an undetermined period of time. Over and over he would get a job and just when I got settled back into doing things I wanted to do he would lose his job and go into a cycle of depression and manic determination to start a business or a new romantic relationship. I never knew what else he would come up with and how I should react or where I should go for help. And, right or wrong, I felt there were very few people who really understood and could help me so I did the best I could to figure it out as I went along.

For families with a child who has had a brain injury there might be ongoing medical challenges that come and go, and some children face behavioral and learning difficulties at school or in social situations. Is it the child's fault he or she can't learn to read as quickly as other students who have not had something happen to their brains? Of course not. But for a parent who sees the child looking the same as before the brain injury it may be frustrating and confusing to find that learning or behavior is different. "Try harder!" they might say to the child. Even without a brain injury no one really knows what try harder means. If those parents live in a place where teachers and doctors understand brain injury, they may get good support and advice. But more often they are told how to control the child with advice that lacks understanding of the brain and the effects of an injury. After doing what the "experts" suggest, parents often become even more frustrated when it doesn't work. All too often these children are labeled as "emotionally disturbed" or "behavior problems" and the parents believe that when in fact their young brains have been damaged in the process of developing and they need special interventions to help them. Parents' hearts break as they watch their child falling further behind the children he or she used to play and learn with.

Many times the cognitive problems that result from a brain injury mean that person, whether a child or adult, can no longer advocate for him or herself. The ability to say, "This is what I need" takes a lot of insight and clear thought processing for most of us, and if someone has trouble organizing his thoughts, or other communication problems, it's too hard. And the rest of the world is too impatient. I have even seen people who profess to be experts on brain injury interrupting someone with a TBI who has to take a long time to speak in a group situation, or not allowing that person to share opinions on a topic just because their thoughts come out a little jumbled. I think the things Jeff says are often profound and worth waiting for, and the same was true with the graduate students who had brain injury and bravely entered the Master's degree program at GW. They offered so much wisdom from their experience that we waited in class if it took a while for them to put their thoughts into words. One of my graduate students, studying to be a special education teacher, said kids with brain injuries should always be allowed to raise their hands when the teacher was talking in class and should not be asked to wait. Why? Because that student might forget his or her question by the time the teacher was ready for Q and A.

I think the hardest part for family members is judging when to help and when to let people with disabilities, including brain injuries, do it themselves. In Jeff's case I had to be involved in so much of his life, and still do, way beyond the point of comfort for him or me. But when I tried to leave it all to him, frightening things happened and so I have had to accept that my role as a parent will always be different than it is with his brother for example. I now know that when he meets with anyone related to his government benefits or anything else where it is important to his well-being, I go with him. I take notes for him and I help him remember follow-up appointments or things to do. Even though he is forty-five years old now, and a parent, he still needs my help. It doesn't fit the ordinary patterns and so I just go with what I've learned from mistakenly helping too much or not enough in the past. But I was fortunate that I had a lot of prior knowledge about brain injury and was a therapist. That is not usually the case and family members may need guidance. The key for helping families is to find trained professionals who know about brain injury; unfortunately most professional fields don't do that very well yet, and insurance doesn't provide help for the family members after the early medical interventions are over.

Maybe if we had more family supports available we would not have as many people turning to substance abuse, criminal behaviors, homelessness, and suicide after a brain injury. I am not going to quote statistics here because this is not meant to be that kind of book and because I'm retired from academia, but it is staggering and sad and unnecessary that so many people do not get the help they need. Our veterans and athletes with brain injuries have recently come into national focus so maybe that will help the cause, but I worry that the important role parents, spouses, and other family members play in helping the injured person get through the rest of his or her life will continue to be overlooked and underserved.

This book was hard for me to write but as I have forced myself to look back in so much detail on life since Jeff's TBI in 1989, I have gone through periods of revisiting the grief and sadness, and then coming to a place of joy that we have all come so far. And I've asked myself what have I learned that I can pass on to readers who might be in the earlier stages of coping with their own situation? I hope just reading some of our story will be helpful, and that my experience can benefit others. So I am going to attempt to do something I am uncomfortable doing: give advice.

I think the things that have been the most helpful to me are what I call ALFIE. There was an old movie in the sixties that I loved and the question posed in the theme song was: What's it all about Alfie? Ed and I have asked each other that question a lot as we struggled to understand some of Jeff's decisions and behaviors. Then we also have to ask: how important is it anyway? Is this problem just Jeff burning a dinner and setting off a smoke alarm, or is his latest decision burning the house down? A sense of humor helps if it's just a burned dinner or the smoke alarm going off. If the house is burning down, metaphorically speaking, it's time to jump in and do something and sometimes it helps to know who to call for emergency assistance.

So here is my ALFIE guide for how to manage life after someone you love has a brain injury. Normally I hate any kind of gimmicky solution books with a cute little acronym, but I'm going to offer it anyway because it's what has worked for me. Take what you like and leave the rest as we say in the world of twelve-step recovery.

A IS FOR ACCEPTANCE. It's important to accept the reality; this awful thing has happened and cannot be undone. I think the healing in my life has always been about struggling to accept reality even when I didn't want to. It's normal to wish for problems to go away and our fantasies to come true, to hang onto hope for a better tomorrow, and to search for ways to fix whatever is wrong. For me, and for Jeff I think, I had to stop trying to force what I thought was best on other people. I told myself I was being helpful when I did that, but I know now that I was just afraid and trying to control the future. At the same time I had to accept my own needs and perceptions to be able to set limits with the people in my life who I now know were not always concerned with my welfare or that of other people I love and want to protect. It's important to accept how you feel, whatever that is. Whether you feel intense anger, grief, fear, or something else that you maybe can't even name, just accept it and know it will change. You are on a roller coaster of emotions and experiences.

L IS FOR LEARNING. Family members need to educate themselves about the brain, not to become experts or therapists but to understand what is happening with the person who is injured, and to help everyone adjust and cope with the new challenges that will come up when you least expect it. Most people don't know much about the brain, brain development, brain function, or what happens when a brain is damaged. I thought I knew a lot about TBI when Jeff was hurt but I found out quickly I did not know as much as I thought, and over the years I have been put in a position of constant learning.

As I keep repeating, and cannot say enough, I believe all professionals in any field even remotely related to education and human services need to learn about the brain. But unfortunately there are still too many fields that do not include any formal training about the brain, even teaching. That always struck me as remarkable because where else is the work of facilitating a process of learning, the job of the brain, more obvious? Someone I used to work with said it's like a car mechanic who has never studied the engine of cars. Teachers need to know about the brains they are teaching, but a typical teacher preparation curriculum is not set up that way, although that may be changing a little now as new brain and learning research emerges.

F IS FOR FORGIVENESS. Starting with forgiving myself, I have deliberately worked hard to forgive people in my life who I felt betrayed me at various points. My parents had serious problems with parenting and knew very little about child development or how to support and encourage someone who is not yet finished growing up, and they were very proud and unable to admit to mistakes. I know enough about their upbringing that I have, most days, let it go and tried to forgive them and understand that they just did the best they could with what they had experienced in their lives. My ex-husband, who I realize looks a little like a shmuck in the early part of this book, is not a bad person. And I know I did my fair share in contributing to our marriage problems. He and I were not right for each other but I kept trying to force it, and maybe we hung on too long so he is now off the hook for my anger, although I'm grateful that we no longer live together and don't see each other too often. When Jeff and Hannah moved in with us in 2003, Steve and his mother began coming for holiday visits every year and staying at our house for up to a week at a time. It was hard at first, but Ed and I were willing to do it because our home was Jeff's home now and he and Hannah needed time with these important family members. One Thanksgiving we hosted dinner for Steve and his mom, Travis and Becky with their son, Jeff's old girlfriend Mimi and her new husband, and Barney's parents who at the time had custody of Hannah's half-sister. It was quite the gathering and I loved it! I began to describe us as "the modern American family."

Over the years I found myself forgiving Steve and we now share love and concern for our adult kids and our grandchildren, and we are able to talk sometimes about old friends and things we remember from our years together. Yes, once in a while I put in a dig; I can't help it. And sometimes he gets on my nerves so Ed and I have an agreement that if I need to talk to him because I'm getting triggered by Steve's conversation or actions I send a signal and we go off to "run errands." We are all an extended family now and so we have had many times, including a celebration of Steve's mother's ninetieth birthday, that were wonderful and a positive experience for all of us.

Forgiveness is not about saying everything was okay or even forgetting what happened. It's about accepting that people are who they are, and for myself I need to accept that sometimes I have to keep certain people at a distance who are not good for me even if they have been important in my life. But I don't have to hate them; I can hate what they did to me or other people I love but the person who did it is just a tormented spirit in my opinion. The hardest forgiveness has been with myself because I still do go back to the "what ifs" and wonder what life would have been like if I had been more clear about who I was and who other people were; would Jeff had been in that car crash? It's a pointless question but I do play with it on rainy days.

I IS FOR INVESTIGATION. When I am confused I know now that it's because I don't have enough information and I need to investigate to find out more before I take action. I need to do some kind of research. Sometimes the research is to find solutions to something, but often it is to go deeper into understanding what the problem is in the first place. I had to investigate Bipolar Disorder, for example, because I wanted to try to figure out what part of Jeff's disruptive behaviors stemmed from a mental health problem we didn't identify for a long time and what were the direct result of his cognitive problems from his TBI. I think he began showing signs of BPD as a young teenager and after his TBI the damage to his brain masked the symptoms for the first two years. Then when he began to recover, and became more active in his life, the patterns returned. For some people it's more important to investigate the effects of a brain injury, to learn what has happened to the person injured, or to seek out resources.

Jeff is receiving most of his support now from the mental health system in our area and not brain injury programs, and for him it is working out. But the mental health service delivery system and brain injury services and supports are all too often separate and there is not much written about the overlap of those two conditions. I think they do go together more than a lot of people realize, and the common denominator is the brain. More and more of what we used to call "psychological" difficulties are being found to have relationships to specific neurological problems. And mental health problems can lead to brain injury. BPD, for example, leads to risky behaviors, such as reckless driving, that can often lead to a brain injury. But in the long run, when someone in the family is causing trouble, what matters most is what to do about it. I used to make the mistake of looking the other way, hoping it would all just magically get better. Now I confront anything I see with Jeff that seems off, that doesn't make sense to me, and he understands that he has to explain it to me. If he doesn't, now he will ask his psychologist for help or discuss my observation in one of his support groups, I don't accept lies or cover ups anymore from anyone, and as Hannah becomes a teenager I think being consistent with that family policy is more and more important.

E IS FOR ENJOYING LIFE AGAIN! I don't think it's helpful to advise people to have fun or be happy in the beginning; it's just not realistic. I was so caught up in my trauma years ago that it was almost impossible for me to enjoy anything, and I felt extremely guilty when I tried. But now I have developed an understanding that if there is a God, he or she put me here to enjoy my life and to do what I can so others can enjoy theirs too. People who are caretakers by nature will naturally put their own needs aside when someone they love has a TBI or other serious illness or injury. That's why I always told my graduate students to not criticize when they were dealing with families of someone with a brain injury. I said they should tell parents of kids coming back to school with brain injuries they were doing a good job with something, and to help them rather than judge them, because I know that was what I needed the most at that time. Too many people direct family members in how to help the brain-injured person without thinking that the parent or spouse, or whoever it is, needs to have his or her own life too, and to be able to enjoy it.

As I finish writing this memoir I have to admit that I am stressed because there is so much I want to say, and so many things I can't include in one book. I want readers to finish reading it with a better sense of understanding how difficult it is for families when someone they love acquires a disability and becomes essentially a different person. One of the biggest challenges people with brain injuries talk about is the loss of self, the feeling of having a certain identity as a non-disabled person and then losing it. And for parents, spouses, siblings, children, or other relatives of that person it is also a huge loss and adjustment that should never be discounted. But it is. I also want readers to understand that the rest of the family matters too. There are so few supports for families going through things like what I have described, and each family has its own unique challenges. We need to do more for families, especially in a country that espouses family values.

If I ruled the world, professional people in all fields of education, psychology, rehabilitation therapies, social work or any other human service would be well trained on how the normal brain develops, and what damage to that brain and its development will do to a child or adult. I would also set up programs and services for family members to either guide them in the daily problems that come up when they live with or help someone after a brain injury. Some people call it case management, some people call it service coordination, but I would like to call it "another frontal lobe."

There are days I feel I have to be the frontal lobes for everyone in our family because Jeff has damage to those executive functions and memory; Hannah is a teenager and so by definition somewhat disorganized, inconsistent, and impulsive; Ed is well-intentioned but pays more attention to sports and the weather forecasts than to what is going on with the people around him. This was an important factor in my decision to take early retirement from GW; I had a full time job at home just keeping our family on track and I loved it even more than I did my paid work. Am I jealous of my former colleagues who have gone on with their careers and are successful? Much as I'd like to say no, I am. But if I try to practice the acceptance I am preaching here; we are all fine. I had multiple possible futures at one time, and it confused me. But I made decisions based on my priorities and my unforeseen circumstances, and this is the future I got. I'm happy with it and love, love, love my family. What better place to put my crusader energies and volunteer work to use than right at home?

There is a quote I like from Mahatma Gandhi that I think says it all, "Happiness is when what you think, what you say, and what you do are in harmony." I have that kind of happiness now.

I hope this book will find its way into some university classes or book discussion groups, so at the end of this chapter I offer up for consideration a few guiding questions to talk or write about, and research more fully, or address in whatever way you want to. And if you want to discuss any of this with me just get in touch! If I'm out for a few days, enjoying the mountains or doing family activities, I will get back to you as soon as I can. And I think I'm going to start blogging too which I expect will be a whole new adventure in itself.

Discussion Questions

1. Do you know anyone who has had a brain injury, or do you have personal experience with brain injury? If you do how does it compare with the story in this book?

2. In this story about one family what do you see as strengths and weaknesses that the family system brought to Jeff's recovery?

3. What changes might occur in a family as the result of a brain injury?

4. What are the needs of the individual members of a family, and the entire family system, during the various stages of recovery and long-term life with brain injury?

5. What national, state, and local resources are available to assist families living with the effects of a brain injury?

6. How do the roles of parents, spouses, siblings, and other family members change when someone has a brain injury?

7. How do you think the culture, religion, or belief system of a family impact the ways that the family cope with a brain injury and how they might become involved in medical care, education, and advocacy?

Acknowledgements

WRITING HAS ALWAYS BEEN my secret passion and I want to thank people who have made contributions to this, my first book, which I hope will be the first of many because I have a lot of ideas and have waited a long time to say it all. I tell people writing and publishing a memoir is like running around town in my underwear. Hopefully my flaws are not too glaring. Thank you to my ex-husband, Steve Bouck, for giving me the okay to publish our story with all of the conflicts between us that I felt I had to include. And yes, I will send you a signed copy!

There are so many people to thank who have supported me along the way in writing this book and in the many ups and downs of life since Jeff's TBI on February 17, 1989. I have to first thank my family because as exposed as I feel publishing this book, it also tells their stories which are very personal. I have to start the list with Jeff for surviving, for being the wonderful son he is and the most loving and devoted Dad I've ever seen to Hannah, his daughter, and for his profound and honest contributions to this book. And for giving me permission all of these years to share our story and his problems and how he has had the courage to work on them. I have to give a special hug and thank you to my granddaughter-daughter, Hannah Bouck, who first of all allowed me to write about her, which for a teenager is a big deal! And for her suggestions as I finished the writing and began to think about marketing. Hannah, you are an amazing gift in my life and I love you. Then there is my loving and supportive husband, Ed Schappell, who came along just at the right time in my life when I needed his particular quirky kind of humor, his undying love and commitment, and the deep friendship we have that has given me the courage to write such a personal book as a memoir. I also want to thank my son Travis Bouck, Jeff's brother, who has been a huge support for me and for Jeff over the years and who is himself a wonderful and devoted Dad to his own son. I'm so proud of our entire family, and extended family, who have all weathered the storm and gone on with life. I also want to thank my friend Monica Rasmussen for her photography skills, and Richard Morales, author and screenwriter, for his valuable suggestions and support as I worked through my fears about publishing a memoir.

I have to acknowledge the work of Sheila Trask in her help as an author consultant with her gentle but wise advice on my messy early drafts and later as a proofreader and copyeditor. The amazing people with the Colorado Independent Publishers Association (CIPA) have given me so much insight into what I needed to do and how to make decisions about the publishing and marketing phase of writing, and I thank them collectively for that. And included in that group of new people in my life are Joe and Jan McDaniel with BookCrafters who have guided and helped me so much in the process of publishing my first book. My dear friends, Betsy Cromwell, Kim Callahan, and Dr. Sharon Montes also helped me by being supportive and insightful beta readers. Having people who are more or less objective read it through was so helpful.

The people who have supported me in my career, especially in the field of brain injury advocacy and teaching/training, are also on my thank you list to thank but there are too many of them to name specifically. If you are not included in my narrative, please know that I do appreciate you and the long conversations we had and work we did together. This includes all of my former students and professional colleagues, and the people with brain injuries and family members who I have worked with in so many different ways. Two people I will always be grateful to for their mentorship in my career, and support with reaching my goals, are Dr. David S. Martin, Professor and Dean Emeritus with Gallaudet University and Dr. Carol Kochhar Bryant, Senior Associate Dean at the George Washington University.

There are many people I cannot list here but their stories have influenced me in choosing the path I did in life and in writing this book. There are other books that offer wonderful personal stories about life after a brain injury, and about other types of disabilities or medical conditions, To find some of these books please see the following web links: http://www.brainline.org and http://www. biausa.org. Those links are also extremely useful to help anyone searching for more information about brain injury, its effects, and resources. For specific information about local resources, you can find the web site of your state brain injury association or brain injury alliance.

Last but not least, all of my readers out in the real world are the most important people in an author's life, so that means you. Thank you for reading my book!

—Janis

About the Author

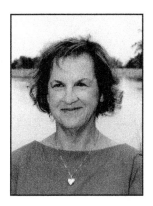

Dr. Janis Ruoff was a speech-language pathologist and disability advocate for over twenty years before her son's TBI and thought she knew about brain injury and its effects, but life after Jeff's car accident taught her how much she did not know until she was living with TBI on a daily basis. She went on to be a leader in the brain injury movement, research faculty member at the George Washington University in Washington D.C., and the founder and Director of GW's Center for Education and Human Services in Acquired Brain Injury.

She lives in Windsor, Colorado with her three generation family. This is her first book. To learn more about Janis and read her weekly blog postings, go to her web site at: www.janisruoff.com.

CPSIA information can be obtained at www.ICGtesting.com
Printed in the USA
BVOW08s2034250916

463265BV00005B/266/P

9 781943 650316